Live Curly, Live Free

Unlocking the Secrets Behind the World of Beautiful Curly Hair

Author: Tiffany Anderson Taylor

ISBN 978-1518702136
Third Edition

DISCLAIMER

The author has done her best to provide accurate and up-to-date information in this book, but cannot guarantee the information has not changed since publication or that it will fit your particular situation. Also, the information contained herein should not be construed, interpreted or regarded in any way as any type of medical diagnosis. **You must always seek help and a proper diagnosis from an appropriate medical professional for disorders of the hair and scalp.**

ACKNOWLEDGMENTS

To my mentor and advanced cosmetology instructor, the talented world champion Michael Della Penna, and his beautiful and equally talented wife, Ellna, who taught me champion-level creative artistry in hair is only possible after mastering the technical skills at the foundation.

To my first beauty school instructor and educational powerhouse, Beth Sheedy, who taught me that the beauty of hair is only as good as the science behind it.

To my clients, who are the kind of dream clients every stylist in the world wants to have.

To my talented editors, Rosemary Anderson, Kim Smith, Jill Terry and Ilysse Weisenfeld, whose hard work ensured this publication was accurate, honest and real.

To my fellow girls with curls, whose willingness to question, experiment, advocate, fight and educate on behalf of the curly hair community everywhere is a proud testament to their collective strength and beauty.

To my parents and siblings, the Anderson family: Will, Rosemary, Robin and Will II. I was blessed to be born into such a fabulous family and I will never know what I did to be so lucky (even if we do resemble the Griswolds).

And to my spouse, Donna Taylor, who always believes in me even when I don't always believe in myself, and who makes my life the most beautiful poem in the world.

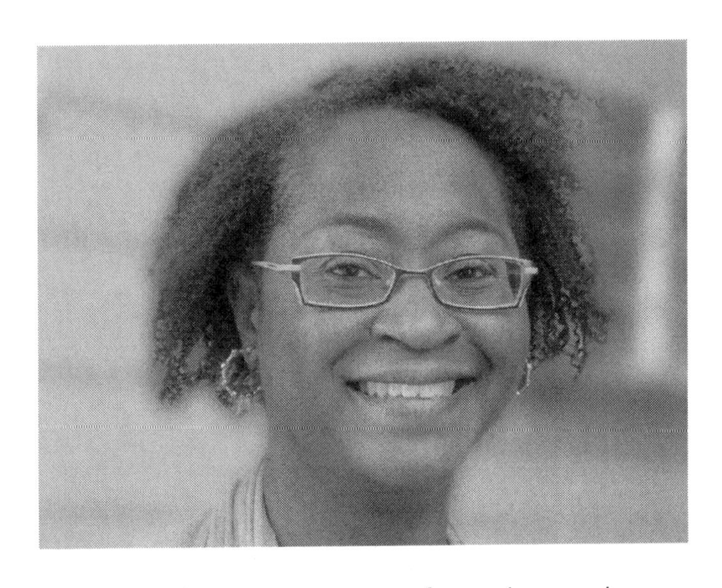

"People always expect more of you when you have naturally curly hair."
- Frieda, Peanuts

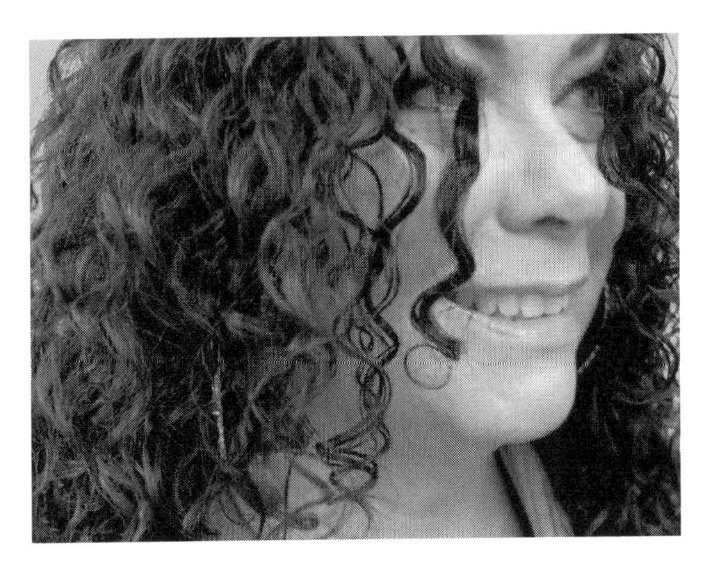

DEDICATION

To my beautiful daughter, Katherine Carolina Taylor, the light and pride of my heart. If I can help you and other little girls to embrace and love your hair in all its natural glory, and spare you all a lifetime of unhappiness and self-consciousness, my precious Katie, I will consider my work a success.

Table of Contents

INTRODUCTION

In 1997, before I became a hairdresser, I moved from Pennsylvania to Florida in late September of that year. The last of the Gulf Coast's brutal summer was behind us, but I didn't know it at the time. The only thing I can remember was thinking how much harder it was to straighten my hair in this subtropical climate. But, although it was much more difficult, it was still manageable, and I smugly figured I had a handle on living life as a "straight girl with curls" 900 miles to the south.

If only I had known.

Fast forward to July 1998. With the onset of Florida's searing and humid summer heat, my hair had morphed from a beaten, dry, yet relatively straight fall of locks into a mess of frizz and cotton wool I couldn't control. I was in a complete panic—whatever was I going to do? I had straightened my hair since I was 16 years old and I didn't know how to live life as a woman with curls.

I cried. I cursed. I spent a fortune on products that promised me sleek, straight hair, but only delivered more of the same frizzy mess. I'm lucky I didn't need an extra room in my beach house to hold all of the products that had been used once and discarded as yet another failure. It was a veritable graveyard.

After about six months of struggle, I finally threw in the towel and took to wearing my frizzy hair scraped back into a ponytail—to work, at home, out shopping, out clubbing, day in and day out. I didn't know what else to do, but I knew I was tired of the battle. I was tired of getting up two hours early every morning to do my hair when I was an unkempt mess by 10:00 a.m. anyway. I was tired of looking and feeling like I had ugly hair every single day of my life.

There was one thing I did know: I loved my hair when it was wet. Right out of the shower, I had awesome, gorgeous spiral ringlets that fell 3/4 of the way down my back. I wished I could figure out how to do them so they would stay that way when they were dry. But it never failed—the more my hair dried, the more the curls would disappear and leave an ugly, frizzy, tangled mess in their place. Most frustrating of all, I didn't understand why.

I found naturallycurly.com not long after its launch and was astounded to find women who had the same problems with their curly hair that I did. None of us had any more insight than the others about why our hair did what it did, let alone how to fix the problem, but it felt good to belong to a sisterhood who "got it"—the frustration, the yearning, the obsession to have beautiful, frizz-free curls, the way nature had intended them to be.

Slowly, over the next several years, information on how to take better care of our curls started making its way to us. I started abandoning "bad" product ingredients in favor of those that were more curl-friendly and was almost immediately rewarded. My hair began to stay more "ringlet-y" and less frizzy. Total strangers started coming up to me to ask to touch my hair and find out how I managed to get my curls to look so good, or even if they were "real."

I was invigorated by the reactions and fired up by the clear need still out there for education about curly hair, so I decided to pursue my lifelong dream of becoming a hair stylist and curly hair expert. Since 2002, I have been studying the science, care and maintenance of curly hair.

After receiving my cosmetology license in 2007, I began passing that knowledge along to a very happy group of curly ladies whom I am blessed to call my clients and friends. They, bless their hearts, call me the "Curl Whisperer" and many of them drive hours, or even fly in from other states, just to come and sit in my chair—primarily because there are so few stylists out there who can handle curly hair properly.

I continue to be amazed at how little information on curly hair is available and at the lack of stylists who know and understand its properties and needs. That upsets me: The science behind the art of curly hair is so straightforward, it doesn't take a rocket scientist to understand it.

Despite the fact that over 65% of the population has curly hair, curl prejudice and ignorance runs rampant through our society (ever seen that television show that pairs wealthy men with attractive women where the "expert" insists wealthy men don't want women with curly hair?). Most beauty schools still place little emphasis on the important differences between straight and curly hair in their educational programs.

Unfortunately, I don't see that trend reversing itself any time soon, so it will take the curly hair community as a whole—both curly clients and curly hair specialist stylists—to promote curly hair education and banish curl ignorance once and for all.

Most frustrating to me is some of the more recent information that leads people to believe their wave pattern has anything to do with how they should care for their curly hair. It makes me crazy to see people buy into the philosophy of "my hair is classified as curl type G52; therefore, I should use products X and Y in my maintenance routine." That is completely wrong and will only spell trouble for the typical girl with curls in the long run.

It is critical for us to understand that the beauty of curly hair is only as good as the science behind it. It is your hair properties, not your wave pattern, that will help you to determine how to care for your curly hair properly. That's basic trichology—good hair science—and in this publication, I'll show why any girl with curls can achieve the curls she wants by first understanding her hair and its properties, then applying a few simple rules to the science of hair so her curls become the amazing, magical things they are and should be.

It is also worthwhile to note that hair science applies to everyone, curly or straight, and can be used even in the event your wave pattern changes over time. My mother, for example, was much curlier when she was younger than she is now—she has morphed into a "strong wavy"—but the principles of hair science are just as applicable to her today as they would have been forty years ago. I personally find it comforting to think that a basic understanding of trichology will allow me to understand my hair for the rest of my life, no matter what my hair decides to do 10, 20, even 30 years from now.

I wrote this publication in a fairly straightforward manner, using plain language—you will notice a distinct lack of fluffy pictures or cute terminology here. You will, however, see **bold type** scattered throughout the pages when I felt a piece of information was important enough to highlight, so pay close attention when you see any bolded text.

There is a lot of information here for you to read and digest, so take your time and don't become frustrated if you don't seem to "get it" right away. Focus on one section at a time and don't rush through it. It isn't difficult, but it will take a while before you completely understand all the principles here and develop a solid familiarity with your new curly lifestyle, so make sure you set realistic goals and expectations for yourself.

I am happy you will be joining me on this interesting journey through Curly World, and I'm willing to bet you will have more than a few "A-ha!" moments as you begin to understand the science of hair as it relates to your own.

Isn't it about time you started to live curly and free?

Tiffany Anderson Taylor
Gulfport, Florida
November 2015

CHAPTER 1 – TRICHOLOGY: THE SCIENCE OF HAIR

Trichology is the scientific study of hair, its diseases and its care. Understanding the structure and composition of hair is absolutely imperative to understanding how certain chemical services, such as texturizing or coloring, or how different product ingredients will affect different hair types. It will be impossible for you to learn how to take the best care of your curly hair unless you understand why it reacts the way it does to certain environments, ingredients and processes.

Understanding Hair Basics

Let's start putting this together to understand how it all works by first focusing on a few hair basics.

What is Hair?

Hair is actually a nonliving fiber made from a protein called keratin. Keratin, in turn, is made up of long chains of amino acids created from what are known as the COHNS ("cones") elements: carbon, oxygen, hydrogen, nitrogen and sulfur. Hair is a dead substance: It cannot breathe and it does not have the ability to directly absorb vitamins and minerals (you must ingest vitamins and minerals orally in order for them to have any beneficial effect on hair health).

The keratin amino acid chains that make up your hair strands are linked together end to end and are also cross-linked together by what are known as side bonds. These bonds are responsible for the strength and elasticity of the hair strand of which they are a part.

There are three types of side bonds: disulfide, salt and hydrogen.

Disulfide Bonds

Disulfide bonds are the bonds that are affected when a chemical service such as perming or texturizing is performed. Your stylist will "break" those bonds and then rebuild them with your hair in its new configuration in order for your hair to go permanently from curly to straight or from straight to curly.

Note: When the hair does start growing out, the new growth will be in its natural state prior to processing, i.e., naturally curly or naturally straight. The texturing/perming or straightening process only will "permanently" affect the hair that has grown out past the scalp at the time of the process.

Salt Bonds

Salt bonds are the bonds that are broken by changes in pH. They are easily rebuilt by normalizing the pH level of the hair.

Hydrogen Bonds

Hydrogen bonds are the bonds that are broken by heat or water. Every time you blow dry your hair straight or use a flat-iron, you break your hair's hydrogen bonds, which will reform with your hair in its new configuration as your hair cools. Hydrogen bonds are also why your hair "reverts" back to its natural state in moist or humid conditions, or when you eventually wash your hair. The moisture in the air and in the water breaks those hydrogen bonds again and your hair resettles back into its natural wave pattern as it dries.

Each hair strand is also made up of three layers: the cuticle, the cortex and the medulla. The medulla is the innermost layer of the hair; however, not everyone has one and it is most commonly found only in thick, coarse hair. When it does exist, it is basically empty air space and any protein that might occasionally be found in it—the importance of which we'll touch on in a short bit—is different from the keratin that forms our hair shaft (*James Robertson, Forensic Examination of Hair, CRC Press, 1999*). The medulla is considered unimportant when it comes to hair services, so we'll only be paying attention to the cuticle and the cortex.

The Cuticle

The cuticle is the outer layer of hair. It is not one solid layer, but instead is made of individual scales that lay against one another just like roof tiles. The cuticle of a healthy hair strand will lie flat and protect the inside of the hair shaft against damage, as well as keep moisture inside your hair where it belongs. Learning how to keep the cuticle of your hair shut is one of the most important things you can do to keep your hair healthy, moisturized and frizz-free.

The Cortex

The cortex is the middle layer of the hair shaft (It is also the innermost layer of hair for those who don't have a medulla). The cortex itself is responsible for approximately 90 percent of your hair's total weight. Additionally, the natural color of your hair is determined within the cortex by a pigment known as melanin. The permanent chemical changes that take place in your hair due to permanent hair color, texturizing, perming, straightening or relaxing take place within the cortex.

One more important part of the equation is the sebaceous glands. The sebaceous glands are the oil glands attached to our hair follicles which secrete an oily substance called sebum. Sebum is what is responsible for lubricating our hair and scalp.

The pH Scale – What It Is and Why It Is Critical to Curly Hair Care

The pH scale is what we use to determine the acidity or alkalinity of a substance. The scale ranges in value from 0 to 14, with 0 being the most acidic and 14 being the most alkaline:

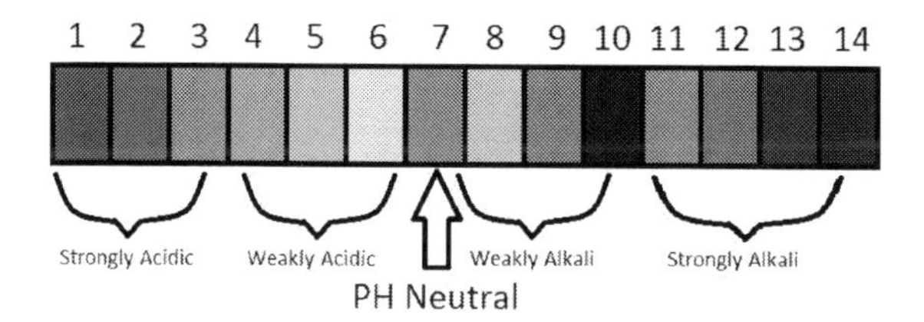

Pure water carries a pH of 7 or "neutral," so anything below 7 on the scale is considered acidic and anything above 7 is considered alkaline. So why is that critical for curly hair?

Remember when I said learning to shut your cuticle is one of the most important things you can do to keep moisture inside your hair shaft and help to keep frizz at bay? Acidic solutions are what shut the cuticle and keep the hair from damage (think apple cider vinegar rinse), while alkaline solutions open the cuticle to let anything penetrate into the cortex (think baking soda clarification). That's why choosing the right products and learning how to use them properly makes all the difference in the health and appearance of your curls.

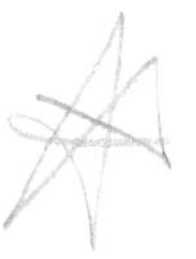

Here is an example: Your hair ranges between 4.5 and 5.5 on the pH scale. Technically, that means even the act of putting pure water on your hair is damaging all by itself because water is naturally more alkaline than hair. That's why you hear so much talk about "acid-balanced" shampoos and conditioners, or why rinsing with apple cider vinegar (pH value 3) or lemon juice (pH value 2) can be so effective. Acid-balanced solutions, when used while cleansing your hair, bring your hair back into balance and shut that cuticle back down!

While the difference between 5 and 7 might not seem like a big deal at first glance, it is important to note the pH scale is what is called a "logarithmic" scale: Each change in number means a tenfold change in pH. So, according to the scale, lemon juice at a pH of 2 is actually 10 times more acidic than vinegar at a pH of 3. And that means water is actually 100 times more alkaline than hair. Looked at in that way, it all of a sudden becomes a very big deal indeed.

Understanding how pH works and how you can manipulate it to your advantage will be a great help in keeping your curls healthy and frizz-free.

Hair Properties

As I mentioned in the introduction, your wave pattern has little to do with how you should care for your particular curls. Wave pattern refers to the amount of movement in the hair, is described as straight, wavy, curly, or extremely curly, and is determined by your genetics or your medical condition. Your wave pattern is completely independent from any other hair properties. While your wave pattern is helpful from a visual identification perspective, it provides little information on the best routine to establish as it does not take any critical hair properties into consideration.

Let me say it again:

VISUAL IDENTIFICATION METHODS DO NOT MATTER WHEN YOU ARE LOOKING TO ESTABLISH A GOOD CURL MAINTENANCE ROUTINE FOR YOURSELF.

So forget whether or not you are wavy or have spiral ringlets, or are classified as "2G" or "16Z" based on some of those "curl classification systems" out there. It doesn't matter. The four main hair properties are the most important factors in hair analysis and they are what you need to know to establish an effective curl care routine, not your visual wave pattern.

The four major hair properties include texture, porosity, elasticity, and density.

Hair Texture

Simply put, your hair texture is determined by the diameter of the hair strand itself. Fine hair has the smallest diameter, coarse hair has the largest, and medium texture is somewhere in between. Your hair texture plays one of the most important roles in how you should care for your curls, not only through daily maintenance, but also when considering any chemical services such as hair color or texturizing. Even how your hair is cut needs to be adapted to the texture of your hair.

There are three different textures: fine, medium and coarse. Not everyone has the same uniform texture over their entire head, however; for example, you can be fine at the nape and coarse at the hairline (especially if those pesky grays are starting to pop up). Let's take a closer look at the different types of hair texture.

Fine Hair

Fine hair can appear very limp or flyaway and does not hold a style well. It frequently seems dry, when in fact it is quite often over-moisturized because heavy emollients (creams, butters, oils, etc.) can easily weigh it down. It is very easy to over-process and is quickly damaged by chemical services if great care is not taken.

Hair with a fine texture does not have the same protein support and structure as does hair with a more substantial texture; therefore, penetrating products (such as conditioners or deep treatments) with a lot of emollients should be avoided in favor of those with protein. Mother Nature didn't give fine hair a whole lot of strength naturally, so the added strength and support provided by protein-based products will help to anchor the hair strand down, and give it a bit more structure, texture and manageability.

Medium Hair

Medium hair is what is considered "normal" hair, meaning it has a mid-range texture. It does not require any special considerations for chemical services and usually processes normally.

Undamaged hair with a medium texture usually has a "normal" amount of keratin protein structure. Those with a healthy medium texture, therefore, generally want to avoid protein in their penetrating products since there is usually little need to strengthen that structure (and could, in fact, lead to over-strengthening issues down the road—see Coarse Hair).

Coarse Hair

Coarse hair is much thicker and stronger than fine or medium hair, but typically does not bend and cannot hold a style well. It is also often dry and brittle because, unlike fine hair, it naturally manufactures an overabundance of protein within itself. Coarse hair is much harder to process and is often very resistant to chemical services.

Since coarse hair carries an excessive protein structure, putting protein-based products on hair that is already protein-heavy will increase the hair structure to the point the hair strand will become just like a broom straw: hard, difficult if not impossible to bend, and very dry. Products that are protein-based should be avoided in favor of those with plenty of emollients, which will help to soften a coarse hair strand and make it more supple (a suppleness it does not naturally possess).

Now that you know what hair texture is, how can you figure out your own?

To determine your texture, grasp a single hair strand firmly between your thumb and index finger and hold it up to the light. Does the hair strand look delicate, a bit insubstantial, somewhat translucent, and seem almost as if it's "barely there"? If any of these characteristics fit, your hair texture is most likely fine.

Does the hair strand look thick, wiry, and sturdy? Does it seem substantial and strong, with a very definitive presence, and is hard to bend? If so, your hair texture is most likely coarse.

Does the hair strand seem somewhat solid, but not overly thick? Does it have some substance to it, but is still fairly supple? If so, your hair texture is most likely medium.

Hair texture is key to establishing the best routine for your hair. As I've said previously, those popular "curl classification systems" that help you in identifying your wave pattern from a visual perspective are fairly well useless when it comes to caring for your curls.

For example: Let's say you and I have the same exact visual spiral pattern, so we both consider ourselves "3B" or loose spiral ringlets. And let's say we both have about the same thickness of hair (density) and about the same porosity, but my hair texture is fine and yours is coarse. Those curl classification systems would still lead us to believe we have the same hair type because we are visually identical, right?

If, however, we try to use the same products because our hair "looks" the same, guess what is going to happen? If we are using products with heavy proteins, my hair is going to look fabulous and yours is going to look like frizzy, crackly dry straw. If we use products with heavy emollients, your hair will look like a million bucks and I'll have a flat, limp, greasy mess. You cannot look to those visual classification systems for information on how to properly care for your curly hair. I know I keep repeating myself, but it is so important to understand that only your hair properties can tell you that.

There is one exception to the rule and that's for hair that's been bleached, also known as "lightened." When you put bleach on your hair, you blow holes in the cortex that look just like potholes. It doesn't matter how "healthy" your hair feels after your lightening service—that only means you have been what we call properly "reconstructed."

Every time you get lightened, you need to have a protein reconstruction treatment to fill in those holes, no matter what your hair texture—protein is not only a strengthener, but it is a reconstructor as well. If you have coarse hair, however, one good reconstruction immediately after the service will probably do the trick, considering you naturally manufacture an overabundance of protein within your hair shaft anyway. Those with fine hair should consider a series of treatments to keep their hair healthy.

Different hair texture types also respond differently to the kind of cutting they receive. Fine hair needs to have a cut with more weight because it tends to lie flat no matter how short it is. Short cuts can be problematic for coarse hair that is very thick because hair with a coarse texture expands naturally in an east-west direction. Even with a curly dry cut, the methodology remains the same, but the stylist has to take all kinds of other factors, including your hair texture, into consideration.

There are special considerations with color as well. The melanin (color pigments) contained within your hair shaft are grouped more tightly in fine hair, so color takes faster and can look darker than expected (because less light is able to reflect through those tightly packed color molecules). With coarse hair, the hair strand has a larger diameter and the melanin pigment is not so tightly packed, so it can take longer to process and can look a bit lighter.

Other than porosity, I would call hair texture the most important hair property there is. Your curly hair care routine will make a huge improvement in the appearance and health of your curls when you start taking your hair texture into consideration.

Hair Porosity

There are a lot of myths out there about hair porosity and how it relates to curly hair care and maintenance. Let's see if we can't set some of the record straight.

Porosity is, simply put, the hair's ability to absorb and retain moisture. Porosity is a critically important factor in determining one's curly hair care. Since moisture is what defines and shapes our curls, the inability to keep moisture within the hair shaft will defeat the most valiant efforts to maximize curl potential.

Hair may not be alive, but a healthy, undamaged hair strand with decent porosity is really good at absorbing moisture. Healthy hair can absorb its own weight in water and can increase its diameter by up to 20%. And since well-defined, frizz-free curls can only form in the presence of healthy, fully moisturized hair, learning how to understand your hair's porosity is crucial.

Further, if you don't know your hair's porosity, you won't be able to make the best product and maintenance routine choices to maximize the amount of moisture your curls retain. The existing curl classification systems never, ever mention porosity in their classification process. Since lack of moisture is one of the biggest causes of frizz, I personally find that odd in the extreme. Just one more reason I don't find those systems very helpful or informative.

Your degree of porosity is directly related to the condition of your cuticle layer. Healthy hair with a compact cuticle layer is naturally resistant to penetration. Porous hair has a raised cuticle layer that easily absorbs water, but is quick to lose moisture as well. Please note that the texture of your hair is not an indication of its porosity. Different degrees of porosity can be found in all hair textures. For example, although coarse hair often has a low porosity and is resistant to chemical services, coarse hair can also have high porosity as the result of damage or previous chemical services.

There are three different classifications of porosity:

Low Porosity

Hair with low porosity is considered "resistant" hair. Low porosity is when the cuticle of the hair shaft is too compact and does not permit moisture to enter or leave the hair shaft. Hair with low porosity is much more difficult to process, is resistant to chemical services, and has a tendency to repel product rather than absorb it. Chemical services performed on hair with low porosity often require a more alkaline solution than those on hair with high porosity, to raise the cuticle and permit uniform saturation and penetration.

Normal Porosity

Hair with average porosity is considered "normal" hair. With normal porosity, the cuticle is compact and inhibits moisture from leaving or entering the hair shaft; however, it allows for normal processing when a chemical service is performed (according to the texture) and will readily absorb and retain product properly formulated for this hair type.

High Porosity (also called Overly Porous)

Hair with high porosity is considered "overly porous" and is the result of previous over-processing or other damage. Other factors that can also affect porosity include heat damage, chlorine/hard water/mineral saturation, sun damage, or use of harsh ingredients. Overly porous hair is damaged in some way, and is dry, fragile and brittle. It has an open cuticle that both absorbs and releases moisture easily; it processes very quickly and can be easily damaged even further if extreme care is not taken when a chemical service is performed.

Although overly porous hair absorbs product quickly, it is often dry as the open cuticle does not allow for product retention within the hair shaft. Chemical services performed on overly porous hair require less alkaline solutions with a lower pH, which will help to prevent further over-processing.

Porous hair accepts hair color faster and permits darker color than less porous hair; however, although overly porous hair takes color quickly, color also fades quickly. While hair with low porosity is difficult for chemicals to penetrate and takes a longer processing time, the color will last much longer.

You can check porosity on dry hair by taking a strand of several hairs from four different areas of the head (front hairline, temple, crown and nape). Slide the thumb and index finger of your other hand down each hair strand from end to scalp. If it is smooth, you have normal porosity. If your fingers move very fast up the hair strand and it feels exceptionally slick, dense and hard, you have low porosity. If your fingers "catch" going up the strand, feel like they are ruffling up the hair strand, or if the hair strand breaks, your hair is overly porous.

Unfortunately, porosity issues stemming from irreparable hair damage cannot be permanently corrected. Only time can truly mend damaged hair. You can, however, create a temporary fix until the damaged part grows out by "reconstructing" the hair shaft with protein treatments. Protein fills in any holes within the cortex (inner layer of the hair) and also helps to fill in the gaps exposed by a raised cuticle.

Individuals with coarse hair, however, must be cautious: Putting additional protein on coarse hair, which is already protein-heavy, can dry it out even more. For those with a coarse texture, acidic treatments such as apple cider vinegar rinses that will shut the cuticle are often a better alternative.

Hair Elasticity

Elasticity is the ability of your hair to stretch and then return to its original length without breaking. It is an indication of how strong the side bonds are in your hair, which are the bonds that hold the individual protein chains of the hair strand into place. More than any other property, elasticity is what dictates your hair's ability to hold its curl, whether natural or created by a wet set or perm.

Normal Elasticity

Hair with normal elasticity can be stretched when wet to up to 50% of its original length and will easily return back without breaking.

Low Elasticity

Hair with low elasticity is brittle, will not return to its original length when released, and usually snaps or breaks easily when stretched. Hair with low elasticity also will not hold a curl from a wet set or a perm.

Previous over-processing and excessive heat styling (flat irons, etc.) are the biggest reasons for low elasticity. I hear a lot of the following from clients who are just starting to let their curls go natural: "I've flat-ironed for a long time and I think my hair has forgotten how to be curly." Hair cannot "forget" how to be curly; only your genetics and medical condition can determine your wave pattern. But if you flat-iron or blow-dry your hair over a long period of time, you compromise the health of the hair by killing the elasticity in your hair strands. No elasticity = dry damage, high porosity and less curl.

To check the elasticity of your hair, wet a single strand, then stretch it to 30%-50% of its original length. If it bounces back to its original length without breaking, you have normal elasticity. If it does not return to its original length or breaks, you have low elasticity.

Hair Density

Hair density is the number of hairs on your scalp per square inch, and is classified as low, medium or high—we usually describe it in layman's terms as "thin, medium or thick." Typically, natural redheads have the least amount of hair strands on their head, about 80,000. Black hair averages 108,000, brown is 110,000, and blondes average the highest density at about 140,000.

Density is important for two reasons: cut and product type. A good stylist will take both your hair texture and your hair density into consideration when determining the most appropriate cut for your hair. On straight hair, for example, someone with fine, thick hair would take a heavily-texturized razor cut well, but using a razor on someone with fine, thin hair will be unflattering since they need more weight, not less of it.

For girls with curls, choosing product type is where knowing your density can be quite helpful. If you have very thick hair, gels—which arc volume-minimizing—are often the best choice in creating a more structured, less "poofy" look. Girls with thin hair, however, will often get much better results by using a volumizing mousse, which creates the appearance of more hair.

So, Now What?

What does all of this mean for the typical girl with curls?

It means this is where those so-called curl classification systems can be problematic. If Type 2 is supposed to mean fine, wavy hair, what happens if you have wavy hair with a coarse texture and high porosity? Or you have tight corkscrew curls often wrongly categorized as coarse, but your hair is baby-fine (as are many curly-hair people with this type of wave pattern) with really low porosity?

If you have wavy hair and follow the routines and use the products normally suggested for this curl type, but your hair is actually coarse and overly porous, you are going to end up with hair like straw—putting protein on top of hair that is already protein-heavy, such as coarse hair, will "reinforce" the hair strand to the point that it will carry too much excessive structure and the hair will not bend (plus, you won't be addressing the problem of your high porosity, which blows product out of the hair shaft anyway).

If your corkscrew curls are fine and you load them up with the emollients often recommended for this hair type, your hair will end up a limp, stringy mess—assuming you can even get the product into your hair in the first place.

It just doesn't work that way.

You need to determine your hair's unique properties, and then think about what types of products are best suited to your particular hair type. Other factors will come into play, but your hair properties are the most important information you'll need to know. Once you've figured out your own hair properties, you will be close to having everything you need to establish the perfect curl maintenance routine for you.

Now that you understand basic hair principles, let's move on.

CHAPTER 2 - WEATHER

Girls with curls have been obsessed with weather and humidity since time immemorial. Will thin hair go flat? Will thick hair get big? Before every major event in our lives, we've studied the weather feverishly, praying it would cooperate enough to give us sleek, beautiful curls (or sleek, beautiful straightened locks) instead of a huge, frizzy disaster. And how often have we been devastated when moisture-laden air has turned some of the most special occasions of our lives into times of tears and unhappiness?

In retrospect, it seems so silly to let something as trivial as our hair spoil major events and occasions. But it's real and it has happened to every single one of us. I know women who look at photographs from events that took place 10, 15, even 20 years ago and still cry over how horrible they thought they looked at what should have been a happy, joyous event.

We all know weather plays a huge role in how our hair behaves on any given day. What most of us don't know, however, is that humidity has little to do with how our hair acts and responds climate-wise. Believe it or not, there are times when the humidity can reach 100% and your hair will be dry, loose and in desperate need of additional moisture. Sounds like a huge contradiction, doesn't it? But for optimum curl behavior, the humidity is the last piece of weather information we need to make informed choices about our curl maintenance routine.

It's not about the humidity. It's all about the dew point.

Every morning at breakfast, Mr. or Ms. Meteorologist is on hand during the morning news to give us the forecast: "... and the temperature is 65°F, the dew point is 57°F, relative humidity is 94%." "Yikes," we think automatically as we munch our bagel and sip our coffee, "94% humidity. Ugh, my hair is going to be a mess."

Only two pieces of weather information battle for supremacy in our mind: the ambient air temperature and the humidity. Dew point registers way at the bottom of our recognition scale, if we even bother to think about it at all. But that's exactly the opposite of what it should be, however, because knowing the dew point is the key to understanding how our curls will behave on any given day.

Just what is a dew point, anyway?

The dew point is, simply put, the temperature to which the air must be cooled in order for it to reach total moisture saturation and any additional moisture must "leak" out of the air. Unlike humidity, it is the true measure of the amount of moisture in the air. For example: If the current air temperature is 69°F and the dew point is 57°F, condensation (and dew) will form if the air temperature is cooled down to 57°F because the air is then saturated with moisture and can't hold any more.

And that's when the relative humidity reaches 100%. But there's more to the story.

Just because the relative humidity is 100%, however, doesn't automatically mean you'll have a bad hair day. That humidity figure isn't an indication of how much moisture is in the air—how high the dew point is. The higher the dew point, the more moisture is in the air; conversely, the lower the dew point, the less moisture is in the air, because cold air cannot hold as much moisture as warm air can.

Think of it this way. Imagine a one-cup measure and a 10-gallon jug in front of you. Fill the one-cup measure completely to the top with water, then fill the 10-gallon jug about two-thirds of the way full. Now, the one-cup measure represents 100% relative humidity because the cup can't hold any more moisture. But so what? If that small one-cup measure means the air temperature is 27°F and the dew point is 27°F, there really isn't a lot of moisture in the air. The fact that the humidity is

100% doesn't mean a thing because the cup just doesn't hold that much water in the first place.

Now, the jug is a different story. Let's say the amount of moisture the jug is capable of holding means the air temperature is 86°F and the dew point is 72°F, relative humidity is 62%. Your first reaction on seeing the 62% humidity might be, "Hmmm, it's not too humid today." I guarantee you if you walk outdoors, however, you are going to feel like you ran right into a wall of wet, humid air. The air is just laden with moisture because the jug is capable of holding so much more of it, and that 72°F dew point tells us so.

You are probably wondering how understanding dew point is relative to our hair. And how can you use this information to make your curls the best they can be?

If the dew point is 45°F or below, then there isn't a whole lot of moisture in the air and you are going to have to throw your curls an assist. Each winter, when the weather gets cold and dry, I get calls from clients who have no idea where their previously springy, moisturized curls have gone—who are these loose, dry imposters in their place??? The answer is to pump up the moisture the best way suited to your particular hair type until the dew point rises. My normal amount of leave-in conditioner often turns to a large palmful on low dew point days.

If the dew point is in the 45°F-60°F range, there is a normal amount of moisture in the air and your hair is usually content with a normal amount of conditioner and styling product. These days are when our more effortless "good hair days" happen most often!

Once the dew point starts to rise over 60°F, it will start to feel humid. The higher the dew point, the more moisture is in the air and the less you typically will need to put into your curls on your own—Mother Nature is supplying a whole bunch of it for free. I use much less leave-in on high dew point days since my hair gets more of what it needs directly from the air itself.

You can also gauge the amount of styling products according to the dew point by doing the exact opposite that you are with your conditioning products. If you are putting a lot of moisture into your hair because it is dry and there is a low dew point, you aren't going to need that much gel or mousse. But if there is a high dew point and you are only using a small amount of leave-in, you are going to up the amount of your styling products because you are most certainly going to need the extra hold.

Once you start paying attention to the dew point and how your hair reacts, you will start to understand and anticipate how your hair will behave on any given day, and you will instinctively begin to know how to adjust your curl maintenance routine accordingly.

Which is exactly where every girl with curls wants to be.

CHAPTER 3 – "TYPES" OF CURLS

While curl pattern may not matter in terms of determining what products to use, the size, strength, and shape of curls is nevertheless fun to observe. Finding and visually identifying your "curl type" can sometimes be half the enjoyment of embracing your curly hair. It is important to understand, however, that there is a big difference between finding your curl type solely for visual identification purposes (or styling routines, which we will touch on later) and finding your curl type because you believe knowing how your curls "look" is the key to understanding how to best take care of them.

At this point, you may also be wondering: If everyone's hair is made from the same protein, includes the same chains cross-linked by side bonds, and is made up of the same cuticle and cortex structure, then why do people have different wave patterns at all?

Surprisingly, we don't really know. One of the most popular theories out there insists the shape of your hair's cross-section is what determines the amount of curl—straight hair has a round cross-section, wavy hair is oval, and curly hair is almost flat. But in truth, that's not always the case. Modern studies have shown cross-sections of hair can be any shape (even triangular!) and they do not always correspond to the amount of curl you have

(*Milady, Milady's Standard Cosmetology, Milady Publishing, 2002*).

A recent and more logical theory proposes that natural curl is the result of one side of the hair strand growing faster than the other side, as determined by your genetics (*Milady, Milady's Standard Cosmetology, Milady Publishing, 2002*). The tension caused in the hair strand will then cause the long side of the hair shaft to curl around the shorter side. Hair with a uniform growth pattern has no tension and therefore results in straight hair.

One of the most significant hair principles to understand at this point, however, is that your wave pattern is completely independent from other hair properties such as texture, porosity, density, or elasticity. One has absolutely nothing to do with the other. As you start understanding more about hair properties, this principle will become quite meaningful when determining the best daily maintenance routine for your curls.

The "Curl Classification Systems"

Several "curl classification systems" have been developed over the last several years in an effort to provide a visual means of identification for individuals with curly hair to determine what "type" of curl they have. A huge ruckus has been made in the past several years over determining what "kind of curl" you have.

It seems, however, that the curl classification systems springing up often do little more than mystify the uninitiated and frustrate others who are desperately trying to figure out a way to categorize themselves. Calls for help abound on message boards as people plead plaintively, "Here is a picture of me ... can you please tell me what kind of curls I have???"

Anyone who knows me can tell you these systems often drive me crazy because they lead people to believe they must take care of their hair based on how their curls "look." The truth of the matter is, they might be interesting and helpful from a visual identification point of view—but, from a stylist perspective, it doesn't really matter what "kind of curl" you have. Not the least little bit. As a matter of fact, trying to force your curls into the tidy little categories ordinarily found in these classification systems is sometimes like trying to herd pigs.

There isn't a curl in the world that will always follow the fixed set of rules that makes it a Type A, a Type B, or whatever. Be honest—you tell me who you know with curls that behave and respond perfectly to their care and treatment 100% of the time just because their owner "knows" they are "Type x" curls. I've had what could be categorized as "spiral ringlets" my entire life and to this day, I can't guarantee you at any given time what they'll feel like doing, even with a virtually identical day-to-day maintenance routine, just because they carry that particular wave pattern.

The only thing—and I mean the only thing—that matters when it comes to the care of curly hair are your particular hair properties: your texture, porosity, elasticity and density. Your wave pattern has absolutely nothing to do with any other hair property. That means knowing if you have "corkscrew" or "spiral" curls, or you are a "5K" or "9T" means a big fat nothing when it comes to the big picture.

Instead, you need to ask yourself: Do you have fine, medium, or coarse texture, or are you a combination of textures? Do you have high, normal or low porosity? Do you have low or normal elasticity? Is your hair thin, thick or medium density? Those are the critical questions you need to ask yourself as you embark on your curly-haired odyssey.

CHAPTER 4 - CURL CARE: CREATING A ROUTINE

It doesn't matter how great of a haircut you have: If you don't know how to care for and maintain your curls at home, your hair will never be the best it can be.

When I was in beauty school, an instructor once told me, "Make sure you never show your clients how to finish their hair as well as you do it, because it will make them think you're a genius." I remember feeling so offended by that. Why in the world would I not want one of my clients to be able to style her hair as well as I can? Why would I not want her to look as gorgeous as possible, no matter who does her hair?

And really, isn't it also in my best interest for my client to look like a million bucks, 24 hours a day? Inevitably, someone is bound to go up to her and ask her, "You have to tell me who does your hair!" That is what is going to make me look like a genius (and, frankly, bring me more business), not holding back on education I firmly believe each and every one of my clients has the right to own.

Here is everything you need to know to keep your curls sassy, healthy and frizz-free.

The Cleanse

There is a whole lot of screaming going on these days about whether to shampoo or not to shampoo. In the last several years, many girls with curls have abandoned harsh detergent-based shampoos in favor of non-sulfate based cleansers or even simple conditioner cleanses in an effort to minimize dryness.

However, advocates of shampooing insist that by not using sulfate-based shampoos to cleanse the scalp and hair, these individuals will start to experience scalp issues and eventual hair loss. These shampoos, they argue, are the only way to ensure the hair and scalp are as clean as they need to be in order to maintain proper hair health.

Piffle, I say. Read on.

What are Sulfates?

Sulfates are harsh, drying cleansers that belong to a class of detergents called "anionic surfactants." They are found in most regular shampoos and are extremely damaging to curly hair because they strip it of its natural moisture, making it frizzy and unmanageable. And sulfate-based shampoos, especially those that include sodium laurel sulfate, can also be responsible for hair loss.

The primary issue with sulfates is that it is very, very difficult to rinse your hair and scalp completely clean of them, leaving behind a heavy detergent deposit—one that continues to build up over time—that can damage your hair follicles. A study published in the Journal of the American College of Toxicology (*Volume 2, Number 7, pp. 127-181, 1983*) cited that hair loss, comedone (blackhead) formation and irritancy can often result from the residue left behind by sulfates.

"Sulfate-free" shampoos have become exceedingly popular within the beauty industry in the last several years. Everything these days is about going green, sustainability and living more organically, so many product manufacturers are now riding that train and marketing their products as more friendly to the environment and to your hair.

Which would be great—except many of these manufacturers are replacing the sulfates with alternate anionic surfactants, such as sodium cocoyl sarcosinate, which we are finding can be just as drying to curly hair as sulfates are.

So I'm going to go even one better on the road to sulfate-free living: I am declaring a moratorium on the use of any anionic surfactant in any hair care product, not just the sulfates, just to make sure we have all of our bases covered (*see "Product Ingredients"*). In the interest of simplicity, however,

I am going to continue to refer to all anionic surfactant-free shampoos as "sulfate-free."

Over the years, it has been my experience that discontinuing the use of sulfate- or other anionic surfactant-based products will restore about 80% of the hair's general health. Now, that's not a scientific number, merely an observation I've made with my own clients, but I don't think there are many sulfate-free advocates who would disagree with me. I'd bet with confidence they've observed exactly the same thing.

Anyone who tells you not shampooing will eventually lead to hair loss is partially right, but they are only giving you half the picture. If you don't cleanse your scalp properly and your hair follicles become clogged with sebum, then yes, you absolutely could start to experience some serious issues. Your hair follicles can suffocate, they can become infected, and/or you can indeed start losing your hair over time.

But it is not the detergents in shampoo that keep your scalp and follicles clean. Movement and agitation are what do the cleansing. Think of a washing machine: That agitator in the middle that swishes your clothes back and forth is there for a reason. Without it, your laundry detergent would be fairly ineffective, no matter how many mountain-fresh chemicals are loaded in there.

If you use a non-sulfate based or conditioner cleanser once a week and give yourself a really good, brisk scalp massage while cleansing—using your fingertips and rubbing your scalp with a firm, energetic circular motion—you are massaging the sebum, dirt and debris out of your hair follicles while stimulating your sebaceous glands to maintain their proper function. The cleanser acts as an agent to carry that oil and debris away without damaging and drying out your hair shaft. That's the real purpose of a cleanser, not this sulfate-based shampoo nonsense that strips your hair of the moisture and oils that keep it healthy.

If, however, you use a non-sulfate based or conditioner cleanser once a week and you squirt a bit on your scalp and kind of halfheartedly move it around, then rinse without really doing any kind of work, you aren't cleansing your scalp correctly and you may, in fact, start having problems. But it doesn't have anything to do with the fact that you are not using shampoo. I've seen clients who use regular shampoo and their scalp is full of dry flakes and scales because they don't cleanse their scalp properly.

I personally believe much of the "you must use shampoo" screaming is an effort to drive more product sales within the beauty industry. Quite frankly, however, if you are doing a weekly non-sulfate cleansing with some serious scalp massage and really focusing on getting your scalp clean, you are doing all the right things and you should never have any issues with clogged or damaged hair follicles (at least not because of your cleansing routine).

The cleansing routine I recommend is this:

1. Apply a sulfate (anionic surfactant)-free cleanser (either a product with a mild, alternative surfactant, or a curly-friendly conditioner cleanser) to your hair and massage it into your scalp for several minutes with a firm, circular motion (don't use your fingernails, just the pads of your fingers).
2. Rinse well with warm water, massaging your scalp to help remove the product.
3. Take a bit more of your cleanser on your fingertips and perform a second, very gentle massage on your scalp—not as long as your initial cleanse, but just for a minute or so. Rinse it out, then proceed with the rest of your routine.

With this dual washing, you've stimulated your sebaceous glands and flushed everything out of your follicles with the first brisk massage (which can also promote hair growth by stimulating the blood flow to the hair follicles), then calmed everything down, relaxed your follicles, and slowed down your sebaceous glands with the second one. I've found this is the most effective way to treat your scalp and it will keep it very healthy.

You should only need to cleanse your hair once or twice a week, depending on the hydration level of your hair. The good news, however, is that if you are using a non-sulfate based cleanser with healthy product ingredients, washing your hair more often should do you no harm if you feel you need to do so.

The Conditioning

Moisture, moisture, moisture! It's all about the MOISTURE level of your hair, my friends. Hair that's been well-moisturized with products appropriate for curly hair and that has good porosity is what leads to healthy, well-defined curls. MOISTURE is what defines and shapes our curls, not product. MOISTURE is what chases frizz away. Curly hair already tends to be dry naturally. Figure in the drying, dehydrating and generally curl-unfriendly products we routinely use and it's no wonder most of us are a dry, frizzy mess.

The biggest offender other than sulfates? Silicones, specifically non-water soluble silicones. If sulfates are Public Enemy #1, non-water soluble silicones occupy second place on the FBI (Frizz Buster Identification) Most Wanted list.

Why Some Silicones are Not Our Friends

Many conditioners and styling products on the market, both professional and drugstore brands, contain non-water soluble silicones, which lie on top of the hair, creating an impenetrable barrier into the hair shaft. They look like a quick fix for frizz since they temporarily smooth the hair shaft down and make frizz seem to disappear—but they also prevent moisture from getting inside the hair shaft, dehydrating curly locks and creating more frizz in the long run. Because they can't be rinsed away with water, they also can build up on the hair shaft and generally require a surfactant-based shampoo to remove. Yet one more vicious cycle in the minefield of curly hair health.

(Remember what I told you about product manufacturers replacing the sulfates in shampoo with other harsh anionic surfactants so they can call it "sulfate-free"? Please be aware they are doing the same thing with silicones these days as well: They are replacing the sulfates in shampoo with silicones so they can call them "sulfate-free" to lead you to believe they are better for your hair. These silicone-laden shampoos, however, will be almost as drying to your hair as a sulfate-based shampoo would be. Don't **EVER** take anything the labels on a product tell you at face value. Please take a few moments to carefully read the product ingredients list on any products you buy to ensure what you are purchasing for your hair is truly a healthy curly-friendly option.)

For well-moisturized, healthy curls, you absolutely, positively must use a conditioner that's either silicone-free or has acceptable, curly-friendly silicones in it (*see "Product Ingredients"*).

To effectively apply the conditioner to your hair:

1. Rake your conditioner liberally all through your hair with your fingers, then comb it through with a pick or a wide-tooth comb, and let it sit for a few minutes so your hair can absorb what it needs. Some methods advocate fingers-only; I find using a comb to finish applying conditioner is more effective for two reasons: a) You will get a more thorough and even product coating on the hair, and b) Any loose hairs will be more easily and thoroughly removed using a comb to rake through your length rather than your fingers.

2. Rinse out any excess with cool water. Cool water, like acid-based products, will shut your cuticle down and help keep all that healthy moisture inside your hair shaft where it belongs.

Pump Up the Moisture

Adding some conditioner back into your hair as a leave-in will help to pump up the moisture in your hair even further.

Note: This is the one place where I find that wave pattern can sometimes make a difference: Not in **what** you are applying to your hair, but in **how** you apply it. As in any product application, however, find and use whatever method you like best and is most effective for you.

For wavy to ringlet/spiral-type curls:

1. Once your hair has been rinsed, bend over and let your dripping wet hair hang free. Gently scrunch out some of the excess water from your hair with your hands, but don't wring it dry. A basic principle in trichology is that "moisture attracts moisture." A wet substance will always be more attracted to another wet substance than it is to a dry substance, so apply your products to clean, wet hair for best results. Hair products normally work much better on curly hair if it is wet when you apply them.

2. Establishing the amount needed by gauging both your hair's condition and the current dew point, rake in a silicone-free conditioner with your fingers from scalp to ends until your hair feels like wet silk. It's lack of moisture that causes frizz, so make sure your hair is getting enough. As you become more familiar with the routine, you will be able to automatically sense how much your hair will require at any given time (some days, you

might not even need any). Let your instincts become your guide.

As an example: My hair is very moisturized and very healthy, so I typically only need to use a dollop the size of a quarter on my almost bra strap-length hair unless the weather is extremely dry. My hair just loves moisture, however—the more, the better—so I routinely use quite a bit more. If you are just starting on your journey to curly hair health, you will find you might regularly need a good palmful at first, but that amount will gradually decrease over time as your hair becomes more moisturized.

For tighter coils:

1. In 1" sections, take a small amount of conditioner and smooth the conditioner over the section, forming a "stick" and squeezing out the excess water as you massage the conditioner over the section from roots to ends. Do not use your fingers to break up the section, but instead, keep smoothing and squeezing until most of the water has been squeezed out of the hair shaft.
2. Repeat until conditioner has been smoothed onto the entire head.

Some individuals advocate just leaving in some of your original conditioner rather than rinsing it all out and applying additional product as your leave-in. I disagree with that approach for two reasons: One, how do you gauge how much you've rinsed out of your hair or know that you've left in enough of the conditioner to be effective? Sticking your head under a shower head or a hand-held sprayer doesn't exactly give you the best level of control and you may be rinsing out more product than you should or not leaving it in the areas where it is needed the most.

Two, most people with curly hair only wash their hair once or twice a week, but many of us do a rinse and condition every day or every other day. And let's face it, we live in a polluted world these days: cigarette smoke, vehicle emissions, manufacturing pollutants—there is a ton of dirt and debris in the air that we aren't even aware is getting into our hair. These particles are going to cling to the conditioner you put in your hair and stay in there if you don't rinse it out. So don't you think you should get rid of all that mess and put in a little fresh conditioner instead?

Speaking of leave-ins: I don't generally have a whole lot of use for most products labeled "leave-in conditioners." I find that they are often only watered-down versions of regular conditioners and since those of us with curls need all the moisture we can get, why bother? A bit of our regular conditioner as a leave-in is often a far superior (and more cost-effective) method instead; however, if you find a curly-friendly leave-in you love, there is no reason you can't use it.

The Hold

Moisture is what defines and shapes our curls, but styling products are what provide the hold. The same rules for conditioners apply to these products as well: dump the non-curly friendly silicones in favor of ones that are curly-friendly, or that have no silicones in them at all, according to your preference.

For wavy to ringlet-type curls:

1. Still in the upside-down position, rake a tablespoon of gel from your scalp to your ends, distributing the product through the length, but concentrating on the area from the roots to the mid-shaft (this guarantees good product coverage on the top of your head, an area not always coated well with product by only scrunching the product into your hair). Don't forget your crown area and the nape of your neck, two areas that are commonly neglected in styling product application: Lean side to side to reach these areas more easily, if necessary.

2. Liberally scrunch a generous palmful of the gel into the length of your hair, starting at the ends. Scrunch and squeeze your curls in a firm, upward motion to your scalp, squeezing out as much remaining excess water as you can while squeezing

in the gel. The water will mix with the product and form a crystalline cast over your curls, holding them in place and preventing frizz from forming until they are dry.

You don't have to use half the bottle, but be sure you are generous with your product application. It is perfectly okay if you dry "crunchy"; we'll be breaking the cast later and releasing the curl, but that cast is important to hold the curls in place until they are completely dry.

For tighter coils:

1. In 1" sections, take a small amount of styling product and smooth the product over the section in the same manner as the conditioner, forming a "stick" and massaging the styling product over the section from roots to ends. Do not use your fingers to break up the section, but instead, keep smoothing and squeezing until the product has been distributed equally.
2. Repeat until styling product has been smoothed onto the entire head.

Blot Dry and Clip

Now it is time to get rid of the excess moisture in our hair and arrange our curls so they can dry with a minimum of disturbance. For very tightly coiled wave patterns, please be very cautious as it is very easy to break up small coils with excessive handling:

1. To remove the rest of the excess water from your hair, use flour sack towels, a cotton t-shirt, paper towels, or baby diapers—any cotton-based, absorbent product that has a completely smooth surface (regular towels, such as terrycloth or microfiber, are too heavy to be used on curly hair. They can cause friction, which will ruffle the cuticle and cause frizz). Repeat the scrunching process, cupping sections of curls in the towel. Scrunch and squeeze them towards your scalp in a firm, upward motion, squeezing out the remaining excess water.

2. Plopping (aka, plunking) is a method in which wet curly hair is "accordioned" onto the head in a concentrated curl arrangement and secured using a tightly tied towel or t-shirt. Microfiber hair turbans also fall under this description (although I am not personally a fan of them as I think they are generally too heavy for curly hair). Many girls with curls opt to plop as the tightly wrapped head towel absorbs extra water and gives hair a jump-start on the drying process while keep curls in an unmovable and untouchable position. You can plop anywhere from five minutes to as long as overnight, depending on what works best for you. <u>Caution</u>: I find that for very fine, very short or very tightly coiled curls, plopping can often be more of a detriment than a benefit, so be careful

should you want to experiment. If you choose to plop (if you don't want to plop, skip to Step 3, below):

a. Take a large towel, measuring at least 16" by 29", and fold it in half on the diagonal so that it looks like a large triangle.

b. Place the triangle on a low flat surface, such as a countertop or toilet seat, with the point, or tail, away from you and the long flat side running horizontally closest to you.

c. With your head upside down, carefully gather your curls in a loose ponytail on top of your head (do not twist them). Now, "accordion", or scrunch the curls up to the top of your head as you lower your head down onto the plop towel. Aim to place the edge of the long side of the plop towel right over your front hair line.

d. Press your head firmly against the plop towel to anchor it to the surface so that it doesn't move, scrunching your curls firmly against the top of your head as you do so.

e. Take the tail of the plop towel with your left hand and pull it backwards to cover the back of your head, covering the nape of your neck.

f. Holding the tail firmly, reach over with your right hand and grab the right-hand point of the plop towel and pull it tightly to the left over the tail so that it is now on the left side of your neck. g. Holding the right-hand point securely over the tail, grab the left-hand point and pull it towards the right side of your neck.

h. Take the left and right points and pull them up and around the sides of your head to the top of your head, then tie them tightly on the top of your head in a knot. Tuck the tail carefully underneath if the excess fabric covering your neck is bothersome.

i. When you have finished plopping, untie the plop towel. Stand up and toss your hair back gently (do not fling your head back!) and let your curls fall naturally to your shoulders, shaking your head gently if necessary.

3. Use the tail of a rattail comb to make sure none of your curls are catching on each other and they are falling downwards without wrapping around each other. If you wear your hair in a part, this is the time to arrange your curls so they are falling the way you want them when your hair is dry.

4. Clip up small sections of your hair on the top and crown of your head to create more volume as your hair dries:

a. Pinch a small section of hair (no more than 1/2") between your thumb and index finger at the root, pulling up slightly to create a "hump", then slide a flat metal clip in at the roots under the curl, holding the clip on its side right up against your scalp. Make sure you keep the head of the clip clear so the clip will not catch your curls and create frizz when it is removed. How your hair looks now is what it will look like when it is dry, so clip carefully to avoid any funny bumps or corners.

b. Place clips on the top and crown of your head—anywhere you would like to create volume. Don't neglect the back of your head at the crown, an area very easy to miss when you are clipping yourself and a place where curly hair has a tendency to go very flat. Use a handheld mirror to view the back of your head so you can easily spot areas that should be clipped. You can pinch the area with one hand while looking at it in the mirror, then put the mirror down to clip it.

c. I sometimes also like to put two clips at the sides right below the temple area to keep those side curls falling in a downward direction, plus it helps to keep my hair from falling into my face while I am air-drying and going about the rest of my morning routine (I can't stand wet hair falling in my face). Once you get used to clipping and find a clip arrangement you like, you can usually clip yourself in less than two minutes.

The Heat is On – Blow-Dry or Air-Dry?

It seems one of the eternal searches for girls with curls is how to dry our hair quickly and most efficiently, without waiting hours (or days!) for our curly locks to dry.

It will be no surprise to many that the porosity of our hair and its texture are what play a major role in determining how long it will take our hair to dry. In general, hair that is finer and less porous has a much shorter drying time; hair that is more coarse and porous usually takes much, much longer to dry completely. Another factor that may also increase drying time is product build-up on the hair shaft that prevents outside moisture from being properly absorbed.

If you have the time in your routine, it is always best to let your hair dry naturally whenever possible, without disturbing the curls, until they are completely dry. If you use a blow-dryer, however, use a diffuser and gentle heat to dry your curls without touching them and without moving the dryer around continually—a surefire way to set yourself up for frizz.

To diffuse your hair with a minimum of frizz:

1. First, dry your scalp. Keep the diffuser aimed at different sections of your scalp for about one minute without moving (use the cool shot to bring down the temperature if the clips are heating up), then move to a different section. Getting your scalp dry is the most critical part of the process, so pay particular attention to make sure you do a good job here.

2. A popular method for drying the length of your curls with a diffuser is one called "pixie curling", which can help avoid the flyaways and frizz halo you can sometimes get with diffusing. To pixie curl and finish drying the length of your hair:

a. Remove the clips when your scalp area is dry. With the dryer turned off, cup a handful of curls with the diffuser and scrunch them almost up to your head, then turn the dryer on low heat.

b. Keep the diffuser on the scrunched curls, without moving, for about one-two minutes, then turn the dryer off again. Gently let down the curls, then move to a different section and repeat.

c. If your scalp gets too hot during the process, use the cool shot to bring down the temperature level, then return to the heat setting. The important thing to remember is that you must turn the dryer off every time you move to a new section.

d. Repeat until your curls are completely dry.

I personally use a combination of air-drying and diffusing to do my hair. After I clip myself up in the morning, I let my hair air-dry while I go about the rest of my usual routine—fixing breakfast, making beds, packing lunches, putting on my makeup, etc. When I'm ready to go and the only thing I have left to do is put on my shirt, I diffuse for about 10-15 minutes to finish the drying process and I'm done.

Who says doing your hair has to take a lot of time and effort?

"Negative Ion" Dryers

Much has been made in recent years about negative ion dryers, whose proponents claim the negative ion air flow will dry hair faster at lower heat settings, resulting in less damage. As of this writing, there is a lot of talk, but not a whole lot of science behind these claims. I have observed that my drying time and the drying time of my clients does appear to be less with a negative ion dryer than with a conventional one, but I can't sit here and claim I've done a whole scientific study to prove it.

These dryers tend to be expensive, so if you are interested in purchasing one, make sure you do your homework and talk to friends who might already own one and can give you their opinion before you make the investment. I use a negative ion dryer in the salon and a conventional dryer at home, and I'm perfectly happy with my results with both of them. It's all a matter of personal preference!

A Word about Blow-Drying and Flat-Ironing Curly Hair

I usually don't "lecture" about things like straightening curly hair because I believe my clients ultimately have the right to make their own decisions about their own hair. But I won't feel I've done justice to the individuals reading this book without a small word on using extreme heat and hair stretching to straighten curls.

It should go without saying that using a blow dryer and/or a flat iron to straighten your hair stretches and distorts your curls, causing dry, damaged hair over time. If you are still straightening your hair all or part of the time, please think long and hard about what you are doing to yourself.

Every time you blow-dry or flat-iron your hair, you compromise the health and elasticity of your curls—resulting in frayed cuticles, split ends, and brittle, porous hair. Ask yourself this question: Why are you spending the time (and money) using good products and healthy ingredients in an effort to restore your hair's luster and health, only to destroy all of your hard work with such a brutal and curl-unfriendly process?

That said, however, if you would ask me if I would prefer someone straightening their hair with heat or with a chemical relaxer/keratin treatment, I would unhesitatingly pick the heat process every time. Although I'd much prefer that "natural" truly mean no chemical or heat processing, I look at it this way: If my clients want straight hair on occasion, I would much rather they use this method rather than put dangerous chemicals into their hair.

You and your curls deserve the best you can give them, but in the end, only you can decide what is right for you.

The Finish

When your hair is completely dry, it's time to scrunch, arrange and finish your curls:

1. If you haven't already done so, remove the clips carefully, then shake your hair gently to set your curls in motion. Bend over, letting your curls fall free, and gently scrunch your curls to break up any crystallized product. You can use a curl-friendly pomade to help scrunch out the crunch and provide an additional level of hold if you'd like. Only scrunch your curls from the underside, to avoid creating frizz on the top of your head.
2. If you would like more volume, "massage" your roots at the scalp with your fingertips from the upside-down position to loosen the hair from the scalp and to obtain more lift.
3. Shake your head and stand up, tossing your hair back gently. With a light touch, arrange your hair so that it falls naturally, then stand back and admire your beautiful curls!

Points to Ponder

As you begin to get used to your new hair care maintenance routine, there are two things you should keep in mind:

Some people report their hair feels "dirty" after moving to their new no-sulfate, no non-water soluble silicone routine. But, please—don't mistake the feeling of hydrated, moisturized hair with dirty hair. We have been so conditioned to shampoo "until it squeaks" that the feel of dry, stripped hair is all we know. Learn to appreciate and love how your hair should feel: silky, supple and full of moisture.

Additionally, your hair may seem to freak out a little bit with the new routine—a halo of frizz may rear its ugly head in the first week or two, leading you to wonder: What am I doing wrong??? Relax! Your hair is having a perfectly normal reaction to your new no-sulfate, no-silicone routine. After years of being stripped of moisture and natural oils, your curls aren't quite sure how to react to all this sudden hydration. It may take a couple of weeks for your hair to regain its health and settle down.

Stick with the routine, no matter how tempted you might be to give it up, and you will be rewarded with healthy, gorgeous, frizz-free curls in the end.

CHAPTER 5 - PRODUCT INGREDIENTS

If there is one question I am asked more often than anything else by girls with curls the world over, it's this one:

What products should I use???

It's the million-dollar question—and it's one that doesn't have an easy answer. Generally, I don't believe in just handing someone a list of products and telling them, "Use this for your product routine." It may be an easy, short-term solution, but ultimately, it really isn't going to do you any good. If the manufacturer goes out of business or changes the product formulation, or if your medical condition changes and your curls change, or if you move to a different area of the country where the weather is different, etc.—how in the world are you going to know what will work for you as a replacement?

It is in your own best interest to learn about your own particular hair properties and, as I am about to describe in this section, gain an understanding of basic hair product ingredients so you will always, always be able to select the appropriate products for yourself. That way, it won't matter where you live, how your hair changes, or what products come and go on the market—you will always be able to make an intelligent selection based on your own knowledge and not just accept what a product manufacturer or someone else tells you is the best choice for you.

My clients will tell you I am not the least bit tied to "brand"—I care more about the product ingredients you use than I do about what brand you use—so always feel free to experiment and use the products that contain the product ingredients that are best for you and your particular curls. I am not much of a product junkie myself, but I still experiment with different products myself occasionally, as I suspect almost every girl with curls will do for the rest of her life!

Below are some major classes of hair product ingredients, a brief description of each class, and the ingredients that belong in that class so you can start to identify and understand common ingredients listed on product labels. Please note that I have only included what I consider to be primary product ingredient classes relevant to this publication, such as humectants, silicones or surfactants; secondary classes such as emulsifiers, thickeners, or UV filters and sunscreens, etc. are not included.

Carrier Oils

Carrier oils are oil extracts from seeds, fruit, vegetables or nuts that are rich hair emollients (moisturizers). They can also be used to "carry" essential oils, which are either too concentrated or will evaporate upon contact on their own, into the hair. Unlike essential oils, they also do not typically have a concentrated scent:

- Avocado oil
- Canola (rapeseed) oil
- Castor oil
- Coconut oil
- Evening primrose oil
- Emu oil
- Grapeseed oil
- Jojoba oil
- Olive oil
- Palm oil
- Safflower oil
- Sesame seed oil
- Shea butter
- Sweet almond oil
- Sunflower oil
- Walnut oil
- Wheat germ oil

Cationic Polymers

Cationic polymers help hair to lay flat and also make it softer, smoother, easier to comb, and less static. Note: Some individuals can experience allergic contact dermatitis, or a hypersensitivity reaction, after exposure to certain polyquaterniums:

- Guar hydroxypropyltrimonium chloride

- Polyquaternium-7
- Polyquaternium-10
- Polyquaternium-11

Essential Oils

Essential oils are concentrated liquids from plants containing the oil of the plant material from which they were extracted. Because of their concentrated nature, essential oils should not be used in undiluted form as some can cause severe irritation, or provoke an allergic reaction.

Below are some common essentials oils used in many hair products and their perceived benefits. Also listed are any commonly known "contraindications" and cautions for that particular oil. A contraindication is a condition in which application of a particular treatment or substance is not advisable. (For example, if someone is allergic to penicillin, that would be regarded as a contraindication for penicillin use, because further use would trigger an allergic reaction).

Please note that the contraindications listed are for informational purposes only and are in no way meant to be a medical diagnosis. You should not infer these oils are safe if a contraindication is not listed. You should always consult a medical professional to address any concerns you may have about the safety of any product ingredient:

- Atlas Cedarwood: Used to treat dandruff, dermatitis, fungal infections, and hair loss. Contraindications: Pregnancy; use in children. Cautions: Can cause skin irritation.
- Basil: Promotes hair growth by stimulating circulation in the scalp. Recommended for oily hair. Contraindications: Pregnancy; use in children and infants under five years of age; long-term use with history of estrogen dependent cancer or endometriosis. Cautions: Can cause skin irritation.
- Bay: Promotes hair growth by stimulating circulation in the scalp. Recommended for oily hair. Contraindications: Pregnancy, anti-coagulant therapy (blood thinners). Cautions: Can cause skin irritation.
- Chamomile: Soothing to the scalp, and retracts inflamed skin cells. Good for those with chemically treated hair or hair that has had a lot of sun exposure or psoriasis. Can give golden highlights. Contraindications: Pregnancy prior to second trimester. Cautions: Can cause skin irritation.
- Fenugreek: Stimulates blood flow to the hair root, and creates stronger, healthier hair. Contraindications: Can alter thyroid hormone balance.
- Grapefruit: Promotes hair growth and is also a known handmade product stabilizer and preservative. Contraindications: Avoid

use while taking Coumarin, an anticoagulant (blood thinner). Cautions: Citrus oils are photosensitive and should not be applied prior to sun exposure; can cause skin irritation.

- ❖ Lavender: Disinfects scalp and skin and can be very effective on lice and lice eggs or nits. The scent of lavender has also been shown to help reduce headaches, depression, anxiety and emotional stress. Contraindications: Low blood pressure, pregnancy prior to second trimester.
- ❖ Lemon: Can give golden highlights. Effective treatment for dry scalp, dandruff, lice and underactive sebaceous glands. Cautions: Citrus oils are photosensitive and should not be applied prior to sun exposure; can cause skin irritation.
- ❖ Myrrh: Use for dry scalp, dandruff, lice, and underactive sebaceous glands. Contraindications: Pregnancy; possibly toxic in high concentrations.
- ❖ Patchouli: Considered effective when used for oily hair and as a dandruff treatment. Cautions: Can be sedative in low dilutions.
- ❖ Peppermint: Helps to stimulate blood flow to the root of the hair and promotes hair growth. Contraindications: Pregnancy; use in children and infants under five years of age; high blood pressure. Cautions: Use carefully if asthmatic.

- Rose: Very conditioning, soothes scalp, and helps hair look and feel smooth and silky. Contraindications: Use in children and infants under two years of age.
- Rosemary: Effective dandruff treatment, promotes hair growth. Contraindications: Pregnancy; epilepsy; high blood pressure.
- Sage: Clarifies the scalp and cleans away impurities. Also a good treatment for psoriasis of the scalp, as well as dandruff. Contraindications: High blood pressure; pregnancy; use in children and infants under five years of age; epilepsy.
- Tea tree: Effective for use with oily hair, and as a treatment for dry scalp, dandruff, lice, and underactive sebaceous glands. Cautions: Can cause skin irritation and aggravate rosacea.
- Yarrow: Promotes hair growth by stimulating circulation in the scalp. Contraindications: Pregnancy, epilepsy, contact allergic dermatitis. Cautions: Yarrow can be photosensitive and should not be applied prior to sun exposure; can cause skin irritation.
- Ylang-ylang: Effective for use with oily hair and as a dandruff treatment. Contraindications: Low blood pressure. Cautions: Can cause skin irritation.

Fatty Alcohols

Because the molecules in fatty alcohols are more oily in nature than those of other alcohol molecules, fatty alcohols are used as emollients in hair care products and contribute a smooth, soft feel to the hair:

- Behenyl alcohol
- C30-50 alcohols
- Cetearyl alcohol
- Cetyl alcohol
- Isocetyl alcohol
- Isostearyl alcohol
- Lanolin alcohol
- Lauryl alcohol
- Myristyl alcohol
- Stearyl alcohol

Note: Fatty alcohols should not be confused with what are known as "short-chain alcohols," which are effective in aiding the dissolution of product ingredients not soluble in water, but can be drying to the hair when used in large amounts:

Short-Chain Alcohols

- Alcohol denat
- Ethanol
- Isopropanol
- Isopropyl alcohol
- Propanol
- Propyl alcohol

- SD alcohol
- SD alcohol 40

Humectants

Humectants promote moisture retention within the hair shaft by absorbing water from the atmosphere, and also slow down the evaporation of liquid. Under ideal conditions, humectants help curly hair to retain its hydration and spring.

In less than ideal conditions, however, humectants can cause a world of problems. In low moisture areas or dry climates, humectants can actually dry the hair out further by absorbing water from the hair itself when there is no moisture in the surrounding atmosphere to be found.

In high moisture areas or wet climates, humectants will force porous hair to continuously "drink" water from the atmosphere until the hair shaft is swollen, bloated and tangled. Both overly dry and overly swollen hair can become frizzy and/or lose their wave pattern due to improper use of humectants.

Depending on your hair type, humectants should not be used in very dry or very wet climates, or when dew points indicate there is too little or too much moisture in the atmosphere:

- 1,2,6 hexanetriol

- Butylene glycol
- Capryl glycol
- Dipropylene glycol
- Erythritol
- Fructose
- Glucose
- Glycerin
- Hexanediol or hexanetriol beeswax
- Hexylene glycol
- Honey (also contains enzymes that produce hydrogen peroxide, which can lighten the hair if the honey is not first heated)
- Hyaluronic acid
- Hydrogenated honey
- Hydrolyzed elastin
- Hydrolyzed collagen
- Hydrolyzed silk
- Hydrolyzed keratin
- Inositol
- Isoceteth-(3-10, 20, 30)
- Isolaureth-(3-10, 20, 30)
- Laneth-(5-50)
- Laureth-(1-30)
- Panthenol
- Phytantriol
- Propylene glycol
- Polydextrose
- Polyglyceryl sorbitol
- Potassium PCA
- Sodium PCA
- Sorbitol

- Steareth-(4-20)
- Trideceth-(5-50)
- Triethylene glycol
- Urea

Petrochemicals

Petrochemicals are by-products of crude oil and are reportedly added to hair care products as moisturizers and protectants. Like non-water soluble silicones, however, they coat the hair shaft, preventing moisture from penetrating into the hair, and can suffocate the hair shaft, leading to damage and breakage over time:

- Mineral oil
- Paraffin
- Petrolatum

pH Adjusters

pH adjusters are used to adjust the acidity/alkalinity balance of hair products and bring them into a more neutral pH range:

- Ascorbic acid (acidic)
- Citric acid (acidic)
- Sodium hydroxide, also known as "lye", the caustic active ingredient in most relaxers (alkaline)
- Triethanolamine (alkaline)

Proteins

Proteins are used to rebuild and reinforce the structure of the hair shaft, and to restore the strength of the hair. Some curly hair types, especially those with a coarse hair texture, are sensitive to proteins, which can cause dryness, brittleness, and decreased elasticity in hair with an excessive protein structure. Proteins are best avoided if any adverse effects are noted:

- Cocodimonium hydroxypropyl hydrolyzed casein
- Cocodimonium hydroxypropyl hydrolyzed collagen
- Cocodimonium hydroxypropyl hydrolyzed hair keratin
- Cocodimonium hydroxypropyl hydrolyzed keratin
- Cocodimonium hydroxypropyl hydrolyzed rice protein
- Cocodimonium hydroxypropyl hydrolyzed silk
- Cocodimonium hydroxypropyl hydrolyzed soy protein
- Cocodimonium hydroxypropyl hydrolyzed wheat protein
- Cocodimonium hydroxypropyl silk amino acids
- Cocoyl hydrolyzed collagen
- Cocoyl hydrolyzed keratin
- Hydrolyzed keratin

- Hydrolyzed oat flour
- Hydrolyzed silk
- Hydrolyzed silk protein
- Hydrolyzed soy protein
- Hydrolyzed wheat protein
- Hydrolyzed wheat protein
- Keratin
- Potassium cocoyl hydrolyzed collagen
- TEA-cocoyl hydrolyzed collagen
- TEA-cocoyl hydrolyzed soy protein
- Wheat amino acids

Salts

Salts are added to hair care products to help remove excess sebum (oil) from hair and as a hair volumizer; however, many curly types find products with added salts—most notably, magnesium sulfate—extremely drying:

- Calcium chloride
- Magnesium chloride
- Magnesium sulfate
- Potassium chloride
- Potassium glycol sulfate
- Sodium chloride

Silicones

Silicones generally end in -cone, -conol, -col, or -xane and are found in many hair products. They are used to coat the hair shaft to provide a smoothing effect, but can build up over time and

dehydrate the hair shaft, depending on th
type.

Silicones that are not soluble in water, will consistently build up on the hair and will require a surfactant-based shampoo to remove include:

- Cetearyl methicone
- Cetyl dimethicone
- Dimethicone
- Dimethiconol
- Stearyl dimethicone

The non-water soluble silicones listed above are the silicones that should always be avoided. Silicones that are not soluble in water, but whose chemical properties allow it to repel further deposit, helping to prevent buildup (although they will still lock moisture out of the hair and require a surfactant to remove):

- Amodimethicone
- Cyclomethicone (Cyclopentasiloxane)
- Trimethylsilylamodimethicone

A note about amodimethicone: If you do an Internet search on amodimethicone, you will find some sites that list amodimethicone as a silicone that is "slightly" soluble in water as long as two additional ingredients are included in the formulation:

Amodimethicone (and) Trideceth-12 (and) Cetrimonium Chloride (as a mixture in the bottle)

The assumption has always been that the inclusion of Trideceth-12 (a nonionic surfactant) and cetrimonium chloride (a cationic surfactant) render the amodimethicone, non-water soluble on its own, slightly soluble in water and it could be considered fine for use.

Turns out that has been a completely incorrect assumption. What the Trideceth-12 and cetrimonium chloride do is render the amodimethicone dispersible in water. Once the amodimethicone is deposited onto the hair shaft and dries to a film, however, it is not water-soluble, will prevent moisture from getting into the hair shaft and will require a surfactant to remove.

Silicones that are slightly soluble in water, but can possibly build up on some types of curly hair over time include:

- Behenoxy dimethicone
- Stearoxy dimethicone

Although not the best choice, slightly water-soluble silicones can be used cautiously and can usually be removed with a baking soda clarification routine (see Home Remedies) or a cleanser containing surfactants other than sulfates.

Silicones that are soluble in water and can generally be considered safe to use include:

- Dimethicone copolyol
- Hydrolyzed wheat protein hydroxypropyl polysiloxane
- Lauryl methicone copolyol

It is also important to note that if any silicone name—including those in the non-water soluble list—has the abbreviation "PEG-nn (with nn representing a number)" or "PPG-nn" in front of it, it is water-soluble, will not build up, and can be considered safe for use.

Surfactants

A surfactant—sometimes referred to as a detergent—is a substance that, when dissolved in water, gives a product the ability to remove dirt from surfaces such as the human skin, textiles, and other solids. There are several different types of surfactants, ranging from harsh to mild:

Amphoteric Surfactants

Amphoteric surfactants are secondary surfactants, similar in nature to anionic surfactants (see below), but are much, much milder and will typically not dry curly hair as an anionic surfactant will:

- Cocamidopropyl betaine
- Coco betaine
- Cocoamphoacetate
- Cocoamphodipropionate
- Disodium bocoamphodiacetate or cocoamphodipropionate
- Lauroamphoacetate
- Sodium cocoyl isethionate

Anionic Surfactants

Anionic surfactants are the major class of surfactants used in detergent, laundry, and hair care products. Approximately 90% of personal care products that foam include some type of anionic surfactant. Anionic surfactants include "the sulfates" and, given their harsh nature and extreme drying properties, are best avoided by curly-haired types:

- Alkyl benzene sulfonate
- Ammonium laureth or lauryl sulfate
- Ammonium or sodium xylene sulfonate
- Dioctyl sodium or disodium laureth sulfosuccinate
- Ethyl PEG-15 cocamine sulfate
- Sodium C14-16 olefin sulfonate
- Sodium cocoyl or sodium lauryl sarcosinate
- Sodium laureth, lauryl or myreth sulfate

- Sodium lauryl sulfoacetate
- TEA-dodecylbenzenesulfonate

Cationic Surfactants

Cationic surfactants, also known as quaternary ammonium compounds, are sometimes regarded as being more irritating than anionic surfactants. While they are added to hair products to improve combability and shine, as well as to provide a more stable emulsion, they can leave a residual film on hair even when it is thoroughly rinsed:

- Behentrimonium chloride or methosulfate
- Benzalkonium chloride
- Cetrimonium chloride
- Cinnamidopropyltrimonium chloride
- Cocotrimonium chloride
- Dicetyldimonium chloride
- Dicocodimonium chloride
- Dihydrogenated tallow dimethylammonium chloride
- Hydrogenated palm trimethylammonium chloride
- Laurtrimonium chloride
- Quaternium-15
- Quaternium-18 bentonite
- Quaternium-18 hectonite
- Quaternium-22
- Stearalkonium chloride
- Tallowtrimonium chloride
- Tricetyldimonium chloride

Nonionic Surfactants

Nonionic surfactants are a weaker and more liquid detergent and are considered the gentlest cleansers:

- C11-21 Pareth-(3 through 30)
- C12-20 acid PEG-8 ester
- Decyl glucoside
- Laureth-4
- Laureth-10
- Laureth-23
- Lauryl ether 10
- PEG-10 sorbitan laurate
- PPG-1 trideceth-6
- Polysorbate-(20, 21, 40, 60, 61, 65, 80, 81)
- Sorbitol
- Steareth-(2, 10, 15, 20)

CHAPTER 6 - PUTTING IT ALL TOGETHER

By now, you have a broad understanding of hair science basics, how weather affects our curls, which product ingredients are the most effective for curly hair and which should be avoided. The next three pages put it all together to show the general guidelines that can be used for product selection based on hair porosity, texture, climate and product ingredient suitability.

It is extremely important to understand that these are just **GUIDELINES** and an initial starting point to assist you in choosing the most appropriate products for your hair type. You must take your own particular hair and its needs into account as well in order to make the best product choices. There are other factors that can come into play, such as health, genetics, medications, etc., and they always need to be considered in your product selection process.

An additional note: In general, I advocate the use of styling gels over mousses and creams, but that's not to say these products can't be effective. I live in Florida and we combat a hellacious, sub-tropical humidity for several months out of the year, so strong gels tend to work better for us down here.

You might want to bear in mind, however, that mousses can often make hair look thicker—a bonus for those with very thin curly hair. And creams can prevent fine hair from looking and feeling weighed down, so these might be better choices for you. Experiment and play with different styling product types until you find the one that works best.

Product Guidelines - Low Porosity Hair

If your hair texture is fine:

- ❖ Avoid anionic surfactants and non-water soluble silicones in all products; use a baking soda clarification and apple cider vinegar rinse combination or non-sulfate surfactant cleanser to remove product buildup when necessary.
- ❖ Avoid heavy emollients and use protein-based conditioners and styling products in your daily routine.
- ❖ Be observant when using humectants in wet climates/high dew point days; watch for excessive drying in dry climates/on low dew point days.
- ❖ Use very warm water or alkaline solutions to open the cuticle to facilitate penetration of product into the hair shaft; close cuticle back down after treatment with acidic solutions.
- ❖ Use protein packs as needed to rebuild and reinforce the structure of the hair shaft, and to restore the strength of the hair.

If your hair texture is medium:

- Avoid anionic surfactants and non-water soluble silicones in all products; use a baking soda clarification and apple cider vinegar rinse combination or non-sulfate surfactant cleanser to remove product buildup when necessary.
- Avoid protein-based or heavy emollient-based conditioners and styling products in your daily routine.
- Be observant when using humectants in wet climates/high dew point days; watch for excessive drying in dry climates/on low dew point days.
- Use very warm water or alkaline solutions to open the cuticle to facilitate penetration of product into the hair shaft; close cuticle back down after treatment with acidic solutions.
- Protein packs and emollient-based deep treatments may be used interchangeably, depending on need, to reinforce damaged hair structure or to re-hydrate dry hair.

If your hair texture is coarse:

- Avoid anionic surfactants and non-water soluble silicones in all products; use a baking soda clarification and apple cider vinegar rinse combination or non-sulfate surfactant cleanser to remove product buildup when necessary.

- Avoid products with protein and use emollient-based conditioners and styling products in your daily routine.
- Be observant when using humectants in wet climates/high dew point days; watch for excessive drying in dry climates/on low dew point days.
- Use very warm water or alkaline solutions to open the cuticle to facilitate penetration of product into the hair shaft; close cuticle back down after treatment with acidic solutions.
- Use emollient-based deep treatments as needed to re-hydrate dry hair and to improve moisture retention.

Product Guidelines - Normal Porosity Hair

If your hair texture is fine:

- Avoid anionic surfactants and non-water soluble silicones in all products; use a baking soda clarification and apple cider vinegar rinse combination or non-sulfate surfactant cleanser to remove product buildup when necessary.
- Avoid heavy emollients and use protein-based conditioners and styling products in your daily routine.
- Be cautious using humectants in wet climates/on high dew point days; watch for

excessive drying in dry climates/on low dew point days.

- Use very warm water to open the cuticle to facilitate penetration of product into the hair shaft; close cuticle back down after treatment with cold liquids.
- Use protein packs as needed to rebuild and reinforce the structure of the hair shaft, and to restore the strength of the hair.

If your hair texture is medium:

- Avoid anionic surfactants and non-water soluble silicones in all products; use a baking soda clarification and apple cider vinegar rinse combination or non-sulfate surfactant cleanser to remove product buildup when necessary.
- Avoid protein-based or heavy emollient-based conditioners and styling products in your daily routine.
- Be cautious using humectants in wet climates/on high dew point days; watch for excessive drying in dry climates/on low dew point days.
- Use very warm water to open the cuticle to facilitate penetration of product into the hair shaft; close cuticle back down after treatment with cold liquids.
- Protein packs and emollient-based deep treatments may be used interchangeably,

depending on need, to reinforce damaged hair structure or to re-hydrate dry hair.

If your hair texture is coarse:

- Avoid anionic surfactants and non-water soluble silicones in all products; use a baking soda clarification and apple cider vinegar rinse combination or non-sulfate surfactant cleanser to remove product buildup when necessary.
- Avoid products with protein and use emollient-based conditioners and styling products in your daily routine.
- Be cautious using humectants in wet climates/on high dew point days; watch for excessive drying in dry climates/on low dew point days.
- Use very warm water to open the cuticle to facilitate penetration of product into the hair shaft; close cuticle back down after treatment with cold liquids.
- Use emollient-based deep treatments as needed to re-hydrate dry hair and to improve moisture retention.

Product Guidelines – High Porosity Hair

If your hair texture is fine:

- Avoid anionic surfactants and non-water soluble silicones in all products; use a baking soda clarification and apple cider vinegar rinse combination or non-sulfate surfactant cleanser to remove product buildup when necessary.

- Avoid heavy emollients and use protein-based conditioners and styling products in your daily routine.
- Avoid humectants in wet climates/on high dew point days; watch for excessive drying in dry climates/on low dew point days.
- Use cold water or acidic solutions to shut the cuticle to facilitate retention of product within the hair shaft.
- Use protein packs as needed to rebuild and reinforce the structure of the hair shaft, and to restore the strength of the hair.

If your hair texture is medium:

- Avoid anionic surfactants and non-water soluble silicones in all products; use a baking soda clarification and apple cider vinegar rinse combination or non-sulfate surfactant cleanser to remove product buildup when necessary.
- Avoid protein-based or heavy emollient-based conditioners and styling products in your daily routine.
- Avoid humectants in wet climates/on high dew points; watch for excessive drying in dry climates/on low dew point days.
- Use cold water or acidic solutions to shut the cuticle to facilitate retention of product within the hair shaft.

- Protein packs and emollient-based deep treatments may be used interchangeably, depending on need, to reinforce damaged hair structure or to re-hydrate dry hair.

If your hair texture is coarse:

- Avoid anionic surfactants and non-water soluble silicones in all products; use a baking soda clarification and apple cider vinegar rinse combination or non-sulfate surfactant cleanser to remove product buildup when necessary.
- Avoid products with protein and use emollient-based conditioners and styling products in your daily routine.
- Avoid humectants in wet climates/on high dew points; watch for excessive drying in dry climates/on low dew point days.
- Use cold water or acidic solutions to shut the cuticle to facilitate retention of product within the hair shaft.
- Use emollient-based deep treatments as needed to re-hydrate dry hair and to improve moisture retention.

CHAPTER 7 – DEBUNKING CURLY HAIR MYTHS

Below are my thoughts on some currently popular "curly hair myths":

Myth #1 – My "Holy Grail" is Just Around the Corner

Many girls with curls get obsessed with finding what is known among us as "The Holy Grail" for their curls—that mythical, miraculous, one-of-a-kind, priceless treasure of a product that will give the worst rain, hail, humidity, sleet and hurricane-force winds known to mankind.

I was on an HG quest myself for eons and there are times I still find myself falling into that trap. Even when I find a product combination that makes me look great 99% of the time, I'll catch myself thinking: Sure, my curls look great, but what if I stop looking now and that one great product—that one single elixir of magical fairy tales—is just over the hill? And what if I never find it because I was happy with "second best" and I stopped looking too soon? It was enough to drive any girl with curls crazy.

It was with a mixture of relief and sadness that I finally came to the conclusion—after doing hundreds and hundreds of curly heads, and studying reams of information on hair type and product ingredients—that, despite our greatest hopes and wishes, that mythical "Holy Grail"

Just. Doesn't. Exist.

Yes, there are products that are great for our hair that will work wonders the vast majority of the time, sometimes even 99% of the time. There are products with ingredients that love our particular hair type—our texture, our porosity, our us impeccable, frizz-free, red carpet curls—the kind that always snap back into perfect shape even in elasticity—and will make our curls look the absolute best they can possibly be.

For a time. But ...

Hair type changes over time. Texture changes, porosity changes, elasticity changes. Weather changes. The chemical composition of your water changes. Hormones change. Medical conditions change. If there is one thing we can count on in the crazy world of curly hair, it is change. And that means no product is going to work 100% the best 100% of the time.

The same product might work almost as great, but from the bottom of my heart I do not and will never believe one single product can unfailingly give you what I call "red carpet curls"—the perfect, rockin' kind of curls that make any Hollywood Alister turn around and think jealously, "I want her hair." Unless you live in an environment and in a body where absolutely nothing changes, the Holy Grail will have to remain the myth it is.

Incidentally, that's why it is all the more important to understand your hair type and your environment and, subsequently, what product ingredients work the best for your particular situation. There might not be a single Holy Grail, but that doesn't mean there can't be a foundational core of products that act in tandem with each other to give you red carpet curls all the time.

Myth #2 – "Ethnic Hair" Has Special Needs

I get a lot of questions on whether or not I know how to handle "ethnic hair" or about the special needs of ethnic hair. And I'm here to tell you there is no such thing. Hair is hair is hair. Period.

Your hair is fine, medium or coarse. Your hair is porous, overly porous, or has low porosity. Your hair has normal elasticity or low elasticity. Your hair is thin, medium or thick. It does not matter what your ethnic background is. Fine, porous, elastic, thick hair is fine, porous, elastic, thick hair whether it is on an African-American woman, a Caucasian woman, a Native American woman, an Asian woman, a Latina woman—you get the picture.

Now, you may have a genetic predisposition to have a certain type of hair based upon your ethnic background. African-American women often have either much finer or much coarser hair, and a much tighter wave pattern than women from other ethnic backgrounds. Asian and Native American women can be so coarse and stick-straight, cutting their hair is a huge challenge because every slice of the shears can leave a visible mark.

There is no guarantee, however, that your hair will follow a certain pattern just because you belong to a particular ethnic group. I have African-American clients with loose waves and coarse texture; I have Caucasian clients with fine hair and extremely tight coils. And that's just the way it is.

That's not to say we shouldn't take pride in ourselves and where we come from, or not seek advice from others who share the same culture as we do! But by realizing that "ethnic hair" truly doesn't exist on a purely scientific level and knowing that our particular hair type is the key to taking the best care we can of our curls—we will always have those red carpet curls, no matter what our ethnic backgrounds.

Myth #3 – Thick Curly Hair is Usually Coarse in Texture

I continue to be surprised at the number of clients who are astounded to find the thick curly

hair they automatically thought was coarse becau
of its "bulk" is actually quite fine in nature.

As with all types of hair, curly hair comes in all textures and wave patterns, but the prevailing belief seems to be that thick curly hair is more often coarse in texture than it is medium or fine. At least in my experience, however, I've found the opposite is true: Thick curly hair—if not altered because of damage or porosity issues—is more likely to be fine or medium than any other texture.

If you are in doubt as to your own hair texture and are having difficulty determining your own, ask your hair stylist for assistance the next time you go in for a hair appointment. What you find out just might surprise you as well.

Myth #4 – "Keratin Treatments" are a Safe Alternative for Straightening Hair

If there is another chemical service that has received as much press, caused as much conflict and drawn as many battle lines as keratin straightening treatments in recent years, I haven't heard about it. I am asked constantly if keratin straightening treatments are as safe and effective as product manufacturers and some individuals within the beauty industry claim they are.

First of all, let's define what they actually are.

Keratin straightening treatments work by mixing keratin protein, the protein naturally found in our hair, with chemicals such as formaldehyde; the mixture is then "sealed" with a flat iron (the formaldehyde is what holds the keratin amino acid molecules together to keep the hair in its new straight configuration). Proponents claim these treatments will loosen or straighten unruly wave patterns and will also get rid of frizz.

Keratin straightening treatments have come under fire in recent months, however, because the original keratin treatments (mostly popularly, the "Brazilian style" of keratin treatments) used large amounts of formaldehyde in their formulations, which resulted in many reports of health issues such as respiratory problems, eye irritation and hair loss.

Because of the bad press around formaldehyde, several companies subsequently began to market their keratin straightening treatments as "formaldehyde-free," leading consumers to believe the health risks reported by formaldehyde use had been negated. Not so, unfortunately. Many of these products were re-engineered to use alternate chemicals such as biformyl or glyoxal; however, these chemical substitutes are members of an organic compound group called aldehydes—a group to which formaldehyde also belongs. "Different" chemicals, exact same scientific performance, exact same health issues.

Also, according to the FDA, any product that contains less than 2% formaldehyde can be marketed as "formaldehyde-free." So many of these "new and improved" keratin straightening treatment products either contained an alternate aldehyde that was just as risky from a health perspective, or still contained actual formaldehyde in smaller amounts.

There is now a new wave of keratin "smoothing" treatments (Notice the name change?) that have come into play recently that claim they really are 100% natural and formaldehyde-free. Really. They use "natural keratin" and other plant-based proteins to infuse the hair shaft for looser, smoother, frizz-free hair that can last up to four or five months. No chemicals, they say: No formaldehyde or any formaldehyde derivatives at all.

The question, however, is this: Can a truly 100% natural keratin straightening or smoothing treatment really deliver straighter, smoother hair without any chemical intervention?

Let's leave the marketing campaigns at the door and visit the actual hair science behind these treatments to see for ourselves if it is possible.

As we mentioned in Chapter 1, hair is permanently straightened or curled by breaking what are called the "disulfide bonds" in your hair—the bonds that are responsible for the shape of your hair strand. They are the bonds affected when a chemical service such as perming or texturizing is performed. Your stylist will "break" those bonds, using a chemical process, and then rebuild them with your hair in its new configuration in order for your hair to go permanently from curly to straight or from straight to curly.

The marketing of these types of products leads consumers to believe the keratin protein infusion is what is responsible for straightening the hair, not any chemical intervention. It is absolutely impossible from a scientific perspective, however, for protein alone to break disulfide bonds to permanently straighten or even "smooth" curly hair for any length of time. That takes chemicals such as sodium hydroxide (relaxers), ammonium thioglycolate (perms) — or, formaldehyde and formaldehyde-derivatives (keratin straightening/smoothing treatments).

At the hair science level, then, it is clear: Keratin protein alone cannot permanently straighten hair. Some type of chemical intervention is necessary to achieve even the smallest change in a natural wave pattern. Keratin in and of itself cannot not straighten; It can coat the hair and give it a shiny, glossy finish, but this is temporary and will not last beyond a few weeks at the most.

So, can a truly 100% natural keratin straightening or smoothing treatment really deliver straighter, smoother hair without any chemical intervention? Impossible, if you look at the actual hair science behind it.

If you are still considering having any of these treatments done, then please be very careful, very vigilant and do your homework before you have any type of keratin straightening or keratin smoothing treatment done. I know the lure of straighter, frizz-free hair is a huge temptation, but you need to decide if it is worth sacrificing the foundational health of your hair, or your health in general.

Myth #5 – Where There's a Wave, There's a Curl

While it is not at all uncommon for curls to "spring to life" and appear curlier when the right techniques and the right product ingredients are used, switching to a non-sulfate and non-water soluble silicone routine or adopting a new curl care maintenance routine is no guarantee that waves will miraculously morph into curls.

There are a lot of factors that contribute to how "curly" your hair can appear on any given day:

your medical condition, your product choice, the level of hydration in your hair, the weather, your maintenance routine technique, the time of year, etc. Curls tend to be springier when there is more moisture in the atmosphere, looser in wintertime when the air is typically drier. I can make my spirals look a lot looser simply by raking my products into my hair as opposed to scrunching them in.

But all the product, hydration, technique, cutting and manipulating in the world cannot change the actual wave pattern of your hair, which determines how curly or wavy it really is. If you are a true wavy, you can sometimes temporarily alter the appearance of your wave formation with your technique, but no product or routine in the world can make you curlier on a permanent basis if you carry a "true wavy" wave pattern.

Sometimes, where there's a wave … there's a wave.

CHAPTER 8 - CUTTING CURLY HAIR

Some curly hair advocates, myself included, are fairly adamant about not cutting curly hair when it is wet. I can't speak for anyone else, but I can give you my own philosophy on why I believe curly hair should almost always be cut dry.

Curly hair is three-dimensional; therefore, it only makes sense to cut it in its natural, three-dimensional state. When curly hair is wet, the curl flattens out and appears much longer than it actually is, making it easy to cut off way too much—and what girl with curls has never had that happen? Also, when curly hair is wet, it is impossible to see each curl as what it truly is: an independent entity that has a unique relationship to the other curls that surround it.

A stylist who understands curly hair knows each curl needs be approached and handled one at a time, so your entire mass of curls will flow with a beautifully fluid motion while allowing each curl to retain its individual and special characteristics (I call the technique I have developed "Cascading"). Unfortunately, I think few stylists nowadays recognize this important principle. Curly hair is so dynamic, however, how can anyone possibly understand how to shape your beautiful, one-of-a-kind curls unless they can see them and work with them in all their natural, individual glory?

When it comes to actual cutting technique, I am a supporter of the curly cutting methodology in which entire curls are removed in an appropriate pattern to remove bulk and create shape depending on the client's hair texture and wave pattern. I have a fundamental issue with other methodologies that only slice or notch into a curl part of the way to remove bulk rather than take the curl off in its entirety.

I believe when curly hair is cut this way, it looks good initially, but as it grows out, little "twigs" begin to sprout as the two different lengths of the curl begin to separate. The more the curl separates, the more product is required to keep it "glued" together. Additionally, the ends of the hair eventually become thin and appear stringy as subsequent cuts continue to notch into the curls, removing even more bulk and making the curls thinner and stringier as they grow out.

I know this style of cut has its supporters who think this is an appropriate way to cut curly hair, but I am not one of them. I've corrected too many haircuts that were done this way on unhappy clients to believe otherwise.

And it goes without saying that any stylist who uses thinning shears or a razor on your curly locks should be tarred, feathered and run out of town!

Finding a Stylist

Curly hair care aside, one of the most frustrating problems for any girl with curls is finding a hair stylist who knows how to deal properly with curly hair. Of all the complaints I hear from clients who sit in my chair, finding a good stylist who loves, appreciates and knows the world of curls is probably at the top of the list. Why, they ask, do so few stylists understand what it takes to cut curly hair correctly?

In my opinion, there are a couple of reasons. First, you need to understand that most beauty schools focus solely on the basics and teach little about curly hair and its special needs. When I was studying to be a cosmetologist (at a reputable beauty school where I received a very good education), the advice I received about curly hair was this: Cut the hair damp instead of wet and don't put as much tension on the section.

Not exactly the most comprehensive curly hair education in the world, is it? 95% of what I know about cutting, styling and maintaining curly hair are skills I mainly taught myself. It's just not a priority in the American beauty education system right now. It's no wonder brand-new stylists are launched into the world without much of a clue.

You can't really blame the beauty schools, however. Their job is to teach a new stylist what he or she needs to know to pass their state board examinations and, as of this writing, I know of no state board that includes specialized curly hair knowledge on their state board exams. Since it is expensive, not to mention impractical, for a beauty school to include subjects in their curriculum that won't be on the state board examination, most of them don't teach more comprehensive curly hair education.

If we ever hope to effect a serious change, then, I believe it will have to be done at the state board level. Once the state boards require more in-depth knowledge on how to handle curly hair appropriately, the beauty schools will change their curriculums to include this education in their programs.

In addition to that, you also need to recognize that sometimes it takes longer to handle a girl with curls than it takes to handle a straight-haired girl. This industry is almost always based on commission, so the more clients you see and the more services you perform, the more money you make.

That means some stylists (not all, but some) are going to treat you just like they do a straight-haired girl because they don't want you in their chair any longer than you need to be. If their commission is $15-$25 on a cut/blow-dry and they can do two straight-haired clients in the time it takes them to do one girl with curls, some of them are going to go for the money and treat you just like a straight-haired girl. It's sad, but true.

To further complicate matters for girls with curls, some of the hair salon "chains" actually have metrics they use to measure stylist performance. In one popular chain, you have exactly 13 minutes to do a haircut. That means you stick the client's head in a shampoo sink for two minutes, use your shears to do a standard 45- or 90-degree layered "wet cut" in 11 minutes, then get them the heck out of your chair.

You miss your metrics often enough, you can get fired. Even if a stylist working at one of these places wanted to take their time and do a proper curly cut, they couldn't. Moral of this particular story: If you have any hope of getting a halfway decent curly cut, think about staying away from the chains. You might be lucky and find someone who can give you an acceptable wet cut in that amount of time, but you'd be pushing it.

So, what can we do?

First of all, one of the best ways to find a curly-savvy stylist is to walk right up to someone whose hair you love and ask who does it. Tell her you are looking for a new stylist and you think her hair rocks. She will usually be quite flattered and will be more than happy to share info about her stylist. Then get a list together of a few who really seem to appeal to you and call for a consultation.

Whatever you do, please don't just call a salon and ask if they have any stylists who know how to cut curly hair. Of course they are going to tell you 'yes.' Instead, arm yourself with knowledge. It is up to you to advocate for yourself and ask questions. You need to know the right questions to ask to make sure the stylist you choose really is familiar with handling curls. Your list of questions at the consultation should include:

- Where did you learn to cut curly hair? (It most likely wasn't in beauty school, so ask them what kind of continuing education classes they took).
- What product lines do you carry/use in your salon that are specific/friendly to curly hair?
- How many curly clients do you have?
- Do you have naturally curly hair yourself?
- Do you typically wear your own hair curly?

If you find one who sounds good to you, schedule a styling session with him/her to see if you like how they do your hair (believe me, many hairdressers don't know how to finish curly hair, so this can be a good indication of how well they handle it). If you like their work and you feel comfortable, then move on to bigger and better things like haircut and color.

The most important thing to remember, however, is that you always have the power to get up from any stylist's chair and walk out the door. There is no excuse to ever let yourself get talked into anything you don't want, whether it be a cut, color or a style—especially if your only reason is that you are worried about what a stylist or the people in a salon will say about you if you do. Give me (and yourself) a break, please. It is never worth crying and dealing with bad hair for the next three, six, twelve months just because you didn't want to say anything or hurt anyone's feelings.

Trust your gut instinct and roll with it—it will never let you down.

CHAPTER 9 - CURLS AND KIDS

What do you do when you've passed it on?

My daughter, Katie—the love and pride of my heart—will be 11 years old in December. Although she is technically a wavy at the moment, she had her mother's curls when she was a baby (Most of which are currently in hiding. They will reappear sometime during puberty, I suspect—just like Mommy's did).

Unlike most children of her age at the time, though, she would tell you all about her "pretty curls" with little prompting. She still always notices others with curly hair. "Look, Mommy," she'll say when we are out shopping and pass a woman with curly locks. "That lady has such pretty curls!"

I can't describe the joy I feel at being able to give her a positive experience about her hair, be it curly or wavy. So many of us grew up feeling self-conscious about our curls and waves, sometimes with mothers or other guardians who simply didn't understand how to deal with it.

Some of us had all our curls shorn off in short pixie cuts for "control"; Some of us had our hair painfully brushed out until we put cavemen to shame. We felt ugly and "different," wondering why fate was so cruel and why we couldn't just look "normal" like everyone else.

The good news is that, as we educate ourselves about how to deal with curly hair, the more equipped we are to pass that education along to our children. The hardest thing to remember, though, is how quickly our children sense and pick up our attitudes if we haven't quite accepted our curls ourselves.

I had a huge reality check myself when Katie was about three years old. I've learned to love my curly hair, but that doesn't mean I don't still have bad hair days or days during a Florida August where I'd trade my left arm for an afternoon of straight, shiny, frizz-free locks. One day, in the thick of the summer heat and humidity, I was fussing and complaining about how I didn't want my curls anymore when this tiny voice suddenly piped up beside me.

"Me either, Mommy."

Talk about a huge smack in the face. The first thought through my mind was: What was I, a supposed curly hair expert, teaching my daughter? How could I expect her to love her hair if I didn't lead by example and show her I loved my own?

It took a while after that for Katie to understand that curls were special and Mommy really did love her curly hair. Today, I don't hide my bad hair days from her, but I am very careful to make the distinction between disliking my curls and disliking how they are falling on a particular day. And she gets it, thank goodness, but I shudder to think how easily I could have instilled a dislike toward curly hair in her, no matter how innocently.

One of the best presents we can give our children in any aspect of life is honesty and knowledge. I think teaching our curly kids how to love their curls while educating them on the realities of their care is a good part of the game plan. And if you are the straight-haired parent of a curly-haired child, it is doubly important you find resources to help you in understanding your child's gorgeous and special hair.

Here are a few tips on how to help your curly child understand, love and care for their beautiful, unique gift:

1. Teach them that their hair is special. I tell my daughter having curly or wavy hair is a privilege and an honor, and that means it takes a little bit more care than other kinds of hair. It is never too early to start instilling pride of ownership in them: I've had children as young as four or five sit in my chair who were already uncomfortable with or disliked their curls.

2. Include your child in the care maintenance routine of their hair. Of course, a child of two or

four isn't going to be able to participate as a child of 10 or 12 can. But it is still important for you to include them in their own hygiene routine at the level where they can participate, and talk about or show them how to properly cleanse, condition and detangle their curly locks.

3. Respect their preferences. As your child gets older, she will start to express preferences for her hair style as a natural part of her growing identity. Do your best to respect her wishes so she feels her input into her appearance is important and valued.

4. Find a curl-sensitive stylist. All the pride in the world won't combat the damage done by an insensitive stylist who exclaims, "Oh my God, look at that hair!" in disbelief. Before you take your curly kid to a new stylist, arrange a consultation with them prior to your actual appointment to determine their attitude towards and sensitivity to curly hair. It only takes one or two thoughtless remarks to cause years of self-consciousness.

I promise you that instilling pride and self-esteem into your beautiful curly child now will save them years of heartache down the road.

CHAPTER 10 - NATURAL HOME REMEDIES

While there are several fine product lines on the market for the care and maintenance of curly hair, many girls with curls are advocating a move to more natural products, including those made at home. There are hundreds of DIY resources for making your own hair products on the Internet, but below are several "starter" recipes you can use if you have an adventurous spirit and would like to experiment.

Apple Cider Vinegar Rinse

There is some debate on whether or not an apple cider vinegar (ACV) rinse alone can clarify the hair; however, it is helpful to bring the hair back into balance after an alkaline solution has come into contact with the hair and will shut the cuticle back down. Repeated use of ACV rinses can be drying, so limit use to once per month at most:

Combine:

1 tablespoon apple cider vinegar
1 cup warm water

Pour the mixture over the hair after cleansing (do not rinse out), then condition as usual. Any lingering smell will dissipate as the hair dries.

Baking Soda Clarification

With some silicone-based products, clarification must be done to remove the product that builds up over time on the hair shaft. Rather than resort to sulfate-based shampoos to remove this build-up, which can damage and dry the hair, a baking soda cleanse is preferable:

Combine:

1 tablespoon baking soda
2 tablespoons curly-friendly conditioner

Apply the mixture to the scalp and massage firmly, then continue to massage it down the hair shaft to the ends. Work it into hair well, then rinse thoroughly with warm water and follow immediately with an apple cider vinegar rinse.

Note: You must follow any baking soda cleanse with an apple cider vinegar rinse. Baking soda is alkaline—meaning it will raise your cuticle and open up your hair shaft. The apple cider vinegar is acidic and will close your cuticle back down. If you don't follow the cleanse with an ACV rinse, you'll be leaving your hair shaft open and setting yourself up for more frizz than you'd probably like.

Chlorine Buster

It is always a good idea to rinse your hair with plain water prior to entering any swimming pool to prevent chlorine water from penetrating into your hair shaft; however, this remedy will help reverse any chlorine damage to unprotected hair.

Combine:

1 egg, beaten
2 tablespoons olive or coconut oil
1/4 cup pureed, peeled cucumber

Massage well into hair from scalp to ends, then cover with a plastic processing cap. Process for 30 minutes hour at room temperature, then cleanse hair with a non-sulfate cleanser.

Deep Conditioning Treatment

No time for a deep conditioning treatment? Right before you go to sleep, rake a good deep moisture treatment through your slightly damp curls. Cover your hair completely with a plastic processing cap and/or a satin sleep bonnet and go to sleep (throw a towel over your pillowcase for extra protection). In the morning, rinse out the treatment, then scrunch in your styling products, style and go. Voilà! A deep conditioning treatment that doesn't take hours from your day!

Essential Oil Blend for Hair Growth

Please note there is no guarantee this oil will stimulate hair growth in every individual. However, researchers from the Aberdeen Royal Infirmary in Scotland published a study of 86 individuals who used this oil for seven months and reported 44% of people in the treatment group had new hair growth compared to only 15% in the control group.

Combine:

3 drops cedarwood essential oil
3 drops lavender essential oil
3 drops lemon essential oil
3 drops rosemary essential oil
3 drops thyme essential oil
1/8 cup grapeseed oil
1/8 cup jojoba oil

Apply several drops of the mixture to areas of hair loss each night, massaging gently into the scalp for 3-5 minutes. Store oil tightly covered and keep away from heat and light.

Contraindications: Avoid rosemary essential oil when pregnant. Cautions: Citrus oils are photosensitive and should not be applied prior to sun exposure.

Hair Detangler

Well-moisturized curly hair is virtually tangle-free, but this recipe can help with the tangles while you are in your re-hydration process. You can keep this in a spray bottle and spray it on in the shower to help detangle your hair while cleansing and conditioning:

Combine:

1 teaspoon pure aloe vera gel
1/2 teaspoon grapefruit seed extract
2 drops grapefruit essential oil
2 drops glycerin
8 ounces purified water

Mix together in a spray bottle and keep in the shower. Spray lightly to help detangle hair.

Cautions: Citrus oils are photosensitive and should not be applied prior to sun exposure.

Honey Hair Conditioner

Honey is a natural humectant that can help restore moisture to dry hair. The antibacterial properties of honey will release low levels of hydrogen peroxide and can lighten the hair, however, so be sure to warm the honey before use; heating it will negate the effects of the peroxide.

Combine:

1/2 cup honey, warmed in the microwave
2 tablespoons olive or coconut oil

Massage well into hair from scalp to ends, then cover with a plastic processing cap. Process for 30 minutes at room temperature, then cleanse hair with a non-sulfate cleanser. For added penetration, sit under a warm (not hot) dryer for 20 minutes.

Lavender Water Hair Spray

The benefits of lavender essential oil in hair care are many—it can help to disinfect your scalp and skin and it can be very effective on lice and lice eggs or nits. In addition, the scent of lavender has been shown to help reduce headaches, depression, anxiety and emotional stress.

Combine:

1 cup purified water
1/2 tablespoon curl-friendly conditioner or coconut oil
1-2 drops lavender essential oil

Combine in an 8 oz. spray bottle. Spray lightly on hair to refresh throughout the day. Shake well before each use.

Contraindications: low blood pressure, pregnancy prior to second trimester.

Oily Scalp Treatment

While most curly women suffer from dry scalp, curly men often do battle with oily hair and scalp conditions. Whether you are a girl with curls or curly guy, the witch hazel in this remedy will act as an astringent and the mouthwash includes antiseptic properties to help with oil reduction.

Combine:

3 tablespoons witch hazel
3 tablespoons natural mouthwash

Apply with cotton pads (only to your scalp); do not rinse. Cleanse as usual.

Olive (or Coconut) Oil Treatment

Olive or coconut oil is one of the healthiest natural ingredients for hair that is extremely dehydrated and brittle. Coarse-haired girls with curls, who historically have the hardest time keeping moisture in their hair, can greatly benefit from the following deep treatment on a monthly or twice-a-month basis (although this treatment is beneficial for anyone with dry hair):

Warm:

1/4 cup olive or coconut oil

Massage well into hair from scalp to ends, then cover with a plastic processing cap. Process for 30 minutes at room temperature, then cleanse hair with a non-sulfate cleanser. For added penetration, sit under a warm (not hot) dryer for 20 minutes.

Tip: You can buy a can of olive or coconut oil cooking spray and use it to spray lightly on hair for shine and frizz control. Be judicious, as you do not want to make yourself oily from using too much. Keeping the spray can at least 10 inches from your hair while spraying will also help to ensure any propellants will dissipate before reaching your hair.

Protein Pack

Some girls with curls, especially those with fine hair, have a tendency to become too over-moisturized with emollients and need additional protein treatments to restore the health of their hair. This is also helpful for lightened (bleached) hair that has not been properly reconstructed after the chemical service:

Combine:

1 egg, beaten

1 tablespoon mayonnaise (the full fat kind, not the reduced fat)

2 teaspoons olive or coconut oil

Massage well into hair from scalp to ends, then cover with a plastic processing cap. Process for one hour at room temperature, then cleanse hair with a non-sulfate cleanser. For added penetration, sit under a warm (not hot) dryer for 30 minutes.

CHAPTER 11 - FREQUENTLY ASKED QUESTIONS

I'm using a shampoo bar 3-4 times a week to clarify my hair and remove build-up. Do you think this is too much?

I know shampoo bars are all the rage these days and, for natural clarification and removal of product build-up, you can't beat them—anything is preferable to using harsh sulfates or other anionic surfactants. I do, however, have a few concerns about possible overuse of this product.

Shampoo bars typically range from 8 to 10 on the pH scale, meaning they are quite alkaline. Alkaline substances will open up the hair shaft, allowing the cleansers to penetrate within the hair shaft to remove build-up. That, in itself, is not necessarily a bad thing; however, it is important to remember that you are stripping your acid mantle every time you cleanse with these bars.

The acid mantle is the very fine, slightly acidic film on the scalp that acts as a barrier to keep bacteria, viruses and other contaminants or chemicals from penetrating the scalp. As an example: One of the reasons that you are instructed to color your hair when it is "dirty" instead of freshly washed is not because the color will take better on the hair shaft—it is so your acid mantle is intact and will prevent the chemical color from penetrating your scalp.

So, if you are over-cleansing with shampoo bars, you are interfering with the natural acid mantle function and leaving a very vulnerable part of yourself exposed. Your acid mantle is there for a reason and it needs to remain undisturbed as much as possible so it can do its job to keep you healthy.

Also, with the nature of these bars, you must follow with some type of a vinegar rinse, usually apple cider vinegar (ACV), which can cause its own issues from overuse. See the question below for more information on ACV rinses.

I personally think using shampoo bars is a great idea, but that using them once or twice a month is more than sufficient to keep the hair and scalp clean, healthy and beautiful.

I do an apple cider vinegar rinse two or three times each week and love the way it makes my hair feel. Is there a rule of thumb on how often I can do this without damaging my hair?

You need to bear in mind that apple cider vinegar (ACV) is an acid—over 100 times more acidic than your hair—and it needs to be respected as such. Acids can and will start to degrade your hair shaft with overuse, so you must be cautious and pay strict attention to your hair's reaction to frequent ACV rinse use.

Depending on your hair texture and porosity, you may be able to support a greater amount/frequency of usage than others can, but you must be careful to judge yours accordingly. If you are doing frequent ACV rinses and are seeing positive results, then your dilution ratio is most likely suited to your hair type.

If, however, you begin to notice degradation in your hair shaft—breakage, frayed ends, dryness, brittleness, or more porous hair—then you need to revisit your proportions and make adjustments accordingly.

What is an acidifying product?

An acidifying product is one that lowers the pH of the hair and brings it back into an appropriately balanced range. Look for citric acid or ascorbic acid on the product label as an indication acidifying product ingredients have been included in the formulation. Conversely, be cautious with products that include TEA (Triethanolamine) or sodium hydroxide, which are both alkalizing agents and will raise the pH of the product.

You can also "balance" your own conditioner by adding a small drop of apple cider vinegar or lemon juice for each tablespoon of conditioner (do not premix, as the solution can go rancid even if the product already contains preservatives). Don't go overboard—you want to lower the pH of the product to an appropriate range, not make it so acidic that it begins to dry the hair shaft.

I see so many different types of proteins listed on product ingredient labels—what are the differences between them and how will I know when to use what type?

Any protein that is animal-based or that has the prefix "hydrolyzed" in front of it is a stronger protein; those such as natural "wheat" or "soy" are the proteins that are lighter. "Keratin" is the natural protein from which your hair is made.

Your hair's condition and texture is a great baseline to determine how much protein you need. If you want to add protein simply because you have a fine texture and you need the extra support, a light protein treatment is fine. If, however, you have damage from sun, chlorine or chemical processes, a heavier protein reconstruction will then be necessary for any real effectiveness.

Curly hair often looks dull and doesn't reflect the light as well as straight hair does; additionally, permanent color doesn't seem to last as long. Are color glazes helpful in adding shine

and preventing permanent color from fading prematurely? And how are they different from permanent color?

I love color glazes and use them often in my own color work. They add a beautiful dimension to permanent color: For example, in the winter, I like to sometimes apply a clear glaze over my dark caramel color which gives my hair enormous depth and shine. In warmer weather, I like to mix a bit of a cool cherry color with the clear for a more "summery" look.

Glazes can help to prevent permanent color from fading since they add another level of "defense" on top of the hair shaft and normally last anywhere from six to 12 weeks, depending on the type of glaze used.

Glazes are mainly semi- or demi-permanent color treatments with a clear or tinted result. They are different from permanent color in that they only stain the outside of the cuticle, whereas permanent color actually results in a chemical change inside the cortex.

Are deep treatments necessary for all curly hair types? What about salon steam treatments?

Deep treatments can be a great part of your maintenance routine, depending on your hair's individual needs. Because I color, I do a deep treatment twice per month—once right after I color, another at the midway point between colorings (at about three weeks), which helps to keep my hair healthy and in great shape. If you do any kind of a chemical process, a monthly or bi-monthly deep treatment can be a good idea.

People with fine hair, however, should be extremely careful since their hair typically needs more protein, not more moisturizers. I seldom recommend routine deep treatments for any of my fine-haired clients, unless it's an initial series of treatments because she is severely dehydrated. An "as needed" protein pack is usually far more effective here.

I don't think there is a point deep treatments are no longer necessary for most people, but I believe there can come a time where they no longer need to be routine. If you don't chemically process and if your hair is healthy, you can do a deep treatment at arbitrary times just when you feel a little extra moisture is needed—such as if the weather becomes extremely dry, if you've been sick, etc.

The jury is still out on those steam treatments; frankly, I've yet to see where paying $$$ at a salon is more effective than what you can do for yourself at home. Boil a pot of water, remove it from the heat, lean over the pot and hold a towel over your conditioner-saturated head to capture the steam for 5-10 minutes—you'll steam your hair and give yourself a great facial at the same time (throw some mint or rosemary leaves in there for a little aromatherapy while you're at it!).

If a salon brags about how well they do perms—does that imply that they should be good at caring for and cutting naturally wavy or curly hair? Or are the two completely unrelated?

From a cosmetologist standpoint, they are completely unrelated. A stylist can give you a wildly successful perm and still not have the slightest idea of how to cut or care for curly hair.

Do sulfate-free cleansers automatically clarify?

"Sulfate-free" does not necessarily mean "surfactant (detergent)-free." For example, many non-sulfate based cleansers contain an ingredient called "cocamidopropyl betaine," which is a surfactant. However, cocamidopropyl betaine is derived from coconut oil and is therefore not considered harsh like the sulfates; however, it will clarify and remove product build-up because it is still a surfactant.

Clarifying is largely necessary for those who still use non-water soluble silicones in their conditioners and styling products.

I've wanted to change a couple of things about my hair recently and my stylist has been resistant to my suggestions. Is it time to look for a different stylist?

The stylist should always do what the client wants in the end, but sometimes, there is a reason for the resistance.

Example: Client A comes in and wants shorter layers. Stylist keeps talking her out of it because Stylist truly thinks the shorter layers are not suitable for Client A's hair/face shape, etc. Client A insists and Stylist finally gives in. Client decides she hates the shorter layers and they make her look awful. So Client A blames Stylist for giving her a "bad haircut."

That happens more often than you can imagine. So, if you really like your stylist, then sit down and have a heart-to-heart talk with her one last time. Make sure she understands you will not be blaming her if she does indeed give you what you want and you decide you hate it.

You can certainly go and find another stylist, but think about what you're risking: You're making big changes with a stylist about whom you know nothing and who doesn't have any history with you on taking care of your curly locks.

What is the normal number of hairs we should lose per day?

For a long time, conventional wisdom said 100 hairs a day was about normal. However, Milady—one of the top cosmetology educational providers and the source on which many state board cosmetology examinations are based—has recently stated that 30-40 hairs per day may be closer to average.

Bear in mind, though, that most girls with curls have a much greater density than girls with straight hair, which makes us seem like we lose an enormous amount of hair every time we get our hair wet (the shower squirrel in the drain!). As long as your hair is not falling out in patches, there should be little to worry about, although you always want to seek the advice of a medical profession with questions about hair loss.

A FINAL WORD

So, there you have it.

There is a lot of information here and I hope I have given you a good starting point for understanding the best way to take care of your curls. The most important thing to remember, however, is that there is no one-size-fits-all routine for everyone. It is up to you to take the information you've learned and apply it to fit your own particular needs and situation.

Learning a new routine can be frustrating at times, so remember to be good to yourself as you begin to digest this new education. Understand that Rome wasn't built in a day and it will take a while before you understand all the principles here and develop a solid familiarity with your new curly lifestyle. Give yourself permission to make mistakes and don't be afraid to reach out for help.

The resources and support systems currently available online have helped many curly women (and men) as they take their first steps toward finally understanding, loving and embracing their beautiful, special curly locks. Seek them out and know that there are a great many communities out there who will be glad to help you out.

From one rockin' curly hair owner to another, I wish you the best on your journey to curly hair freedom.

ABOUT THE AUTHOR

Called "The Curl Whisperer" by her clients, Tiffany Anderson Taylor—the owner and creator of Live Curly Live Free—is a master hair stylist and curly hair expert located in the Tampa Bay area of Florida.

As a girl with curls herself, she knows firsthand the problems associated with curly hair because she's battled the same problems her entire life. And, unlike many stylists, she understands the importance of cutting curly hair dry so the curls retain their individuality, knows certain ingredients in most common shampoos and conditioners are a recipe for disaster for curly hair, and believes virtually anyone can learn to style their curls so they are soft and flowing—not wet and crunchy—and will hold their shape without frizz.

Girls with curls from as far away as Tallahassee, Pensacola, Jacksonville, Boca Raton and Ocala drive hours to see Tiffany (and even fly in from other states) for, as one curly client put it, "the best hair I've ever had in my entire life." The glowing reviews she has received on curly hair forums on her work and the many referrals she receives from her clientele attest to her considerable knowledge about curly hair, and has earned her numerous kudos on her unique and unprecedented blend of cutting, styling and product education.

Learn more at www.livecurlylivefree.com.

You can schedule an appointment with the Live Curly Live Free salon by calling:

Live Curly Live Free
2914 Beach Boulevard South
The Art Village Courtyard
Gulfport, FL 33707
727.323.CURL (2875)

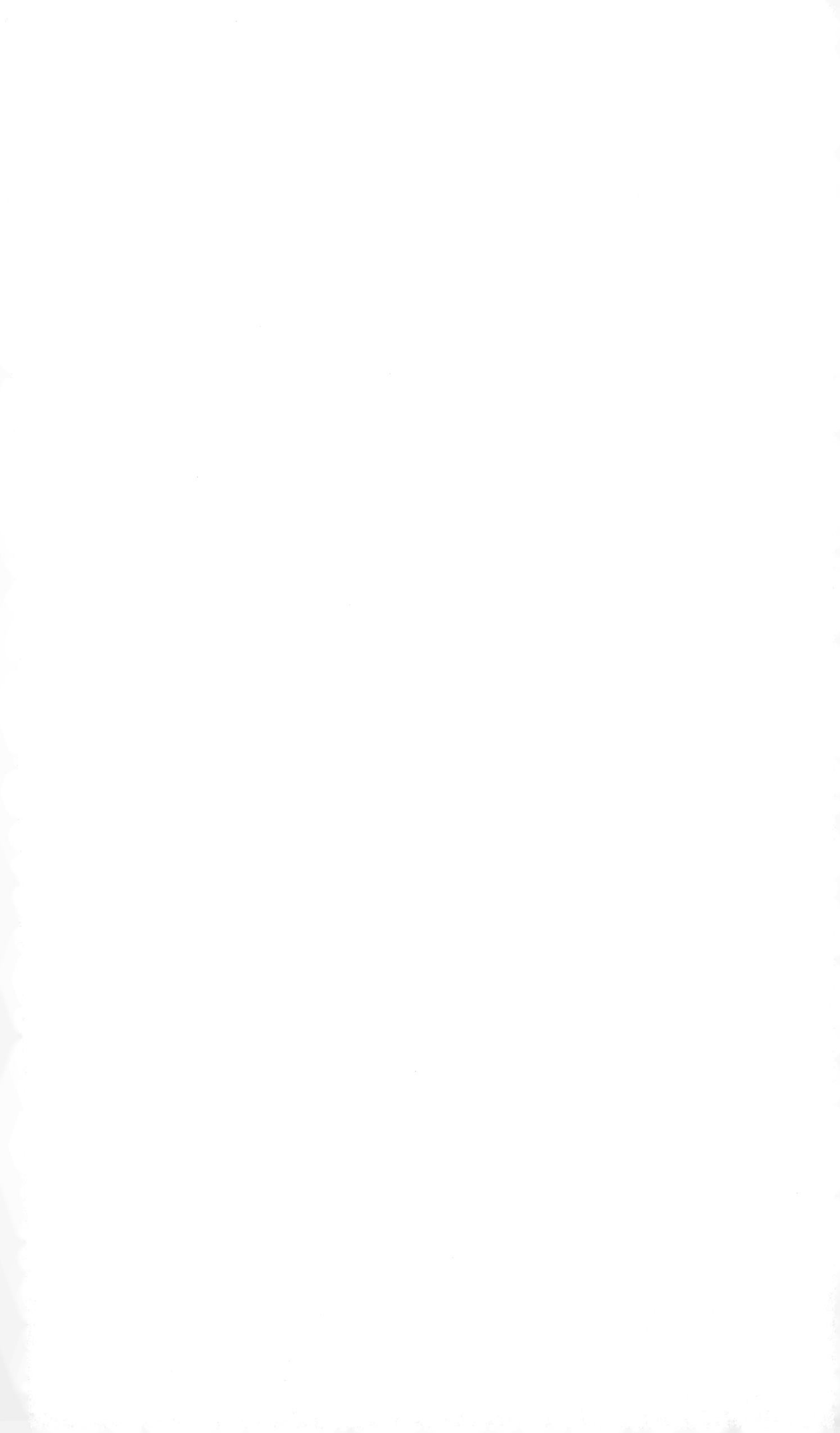

Made in the USA
Lexington, KY
02 February 2019